BIG
yoga.
For Less Stress

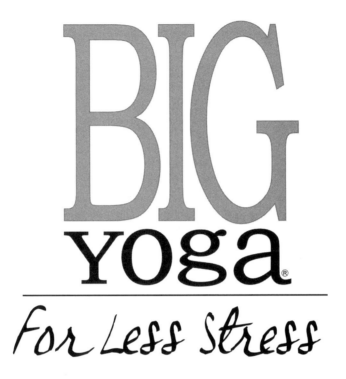

BIG
yoga®
For Less Stress

MEERA PATRICIA KERR

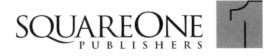

SQUAREONE
PUBLISHERS

As with any exercise program, consult with your doctor before beginning if you have questions or concerns. It is always better to err on the side of caution.

COVER DESIGNER: Jeannie Tudor
TYPESETTER: Gary A. Rosenberg
COVER AND INTERIOR PHOTO CREDIT: Tim LaDuke of LaDuke Studios
(www.ladukestudios.com)

Square One Publishers
115 Herricks Road
Garden City Park, NY 11040
(516) 535-2010 • (877) 900-BOOK
www.squareonepublishers.com

Library of Congress Cataloging-in-Publication Data

Kerr, Meera Patricia.
   Big yoga for less stress : a simple guide to reducing everyday anxiety /
Meera Patricia Kerr.
     pages cm
   ISBN 978-0-7570-0405-6
   1. Yoga—Therapeutic use. 2. Stress management. 3. Anxiety—Exercise
therapy. I. Title.
   RM727.Y64K47   2015
   613.7'046—dc23
                                                        2014046024

Printed in the United States of America

10   9   8   7   6   5   4   3   2   1

Contents

For Sukarta and David,
who know my sorrow
and carry on.

Acknowledgments

After I finished my first Big Yoga book, I found myself at loose ends, working several part-time jobs to keep my not-so-profitable cottage rental business afloat and losing focus on my own personal yoga practice. I had an idea for writing a book about stress management when I was blindsided by the death of my son Sam. If it hadn't been for the the healing practices of Yoga and the encouragement, patience, and kindness of my publisher, Rudy Shur, this project would never have come to fruition.

So many dear ones gathered me into their compassionate arms: Deepa McNulti, who went immediately to the house to look after Sam's dad and brother; Christine McMahan, who came to California to rescue and grieve with me; my Michigan neighbors Mary Anne Wengel, Judy Covey, Jean Birky, Edie Clark, Al Weener, Michaele and Tom Landon, Molly Miller, and Nancy Bruusma and all the children and staff at the Glenn School. Their loving kindness gave me the strength to carry on.

When I finished the manuscript, it was my editor, Miye Bromberg, who shook out the wrinkles and made it into something that I think you'll find easy to use in your practice. Thanks to photographer Tim La Duke, who was generous with his time and talent, and to Gary Rosenberg and Jeannie Tudor, who artfully assembled the manuscript, magically getting all the photographs in just the right places.

My healing has been ongoing, and I have received tremendous support from my dear sangha at the Satchidananda Ashram at Yogaville. Special thanks to my movement mentor, Hope Mell, who continues to reveal the secrets of the Yoga-body, and to Mukunda Stiles, who brought us the invaluable joint freeing series.

Thanks to my son David, for staying strong, and to his homies—John-Liam, Alec, and Miles—who made me laugh intermittently during the worst of my tears.

Finally, I offer my humble gratitude to Sri Gurudev, Master Sivananda, and the ancient teachings of the lineage. Om shanti.

Big Yoga For Less Stress

Introduction

Are you feeling exhausted and overwhelmed? Are you having a hard time juggling work, family, friends, and other responsibilities? Have you noticed that your friends are complaining that they feel overworked, underappreciated, or just plain fried? Time seems to be speeding up, making it impossible to accomplish everything on the to-do list in twenty-four hours.

Stress has become a fact of modern life—we all suffer from it in one way or another. And our suffering isn't just in our heads. A recent study found that while 73 percent of all subjects experienced psychological symptoms as a result of stress, 77 percent also regularly experienced physical symptoms. Moreover, half of the people interviewed felt that their stress levels had increased over the last five years.

Yoga can help. Through Yoga, you can bring your mind and body into balance, allowing new clarity and peace to enter your life. Once your mind is calm and present, you'll find that you're better able to handle any challenge that comes your way. Instead of viewing these challenges as stressors, you'll start to see them as opportunities for growth and positive change.

> "We can be serene even in the midst of calamities and, by our serenity, make others more tranquil. Serenity is contagious."
> –Swami Satchidananda

I was introduced to Yoga in a less stressful time. When I signed up for a Yoga teacher training course back in 1978, rents were lower and gas was cheaper. I could afford to be a hippie, to take a month off from my music gigs and not go broke.

But the techniques I learned under the guidance of Sri Swami Satchidananda have served me well throughout my life. While I was writing this book, my son, Sam, died at the age of thirty-one. The death of a loved one is perhaps the most traumatic event a person can endure. Suddenly, I was forced to put my own practices to the test, using the stress management techniques I was writing about to help soothe my grief. And while I'm still healing, I know that my loss would

have been much more painful if I hadn't had the principles of Big Yoga at my
disposal.

WHY DO WE CALL IT "BIG YOGA"?

You may be wondering, what does twisting myself into a pretzel have to do with
stress management? So often that's how we see Yoga portrayed in the media—
as a feat of flexibility and strength, usually performed by young, lithe athletes.
These images can be deceiving. Remember, the models in those pictures are professionals who may be able to practice the physical postures for several hours
every day!

I'm here to tell you that Yoga can be done by anyone. In my first book, *Big
Yoga*, I adapted the basic techniques of Integral Yoga so that they could be enjoyed
by people of all shapes of sizes. Whether you're slender or plump, stiff or flexible,
young or old, everyone can benefit from Yoga. Yoga is more about a feeling of
wholeness and contentment than it is about getting washboard abs and buns of
steel.

But Big Yoga isn't just Yoga for big people, either. Big Yoga goes beyond the
exercises most people associate with Yoga—that's what makes it big! Big Yoga
encompasses a whole range of physical and mental practices that can calm your
mind and refresh your body: movement, breathing exercises, meditation, chanting, and community service. With all these different techniques available to you,
it will be easy to incorporate at least one into your daily life to help you lessen
your burdens.

HOW TO USE THIS BOOK

Consider this book your manual for stress management. In it, you'll find all the
tools you need to break the stress cycle, allowing you to attain a greater sense of
peace than any you may have experienced before. I've also included practices
that will help you address your emotions, eliciting feelings of joy, cheerfulness,
and hope instead of sorrow, depression, and despair.

Part One provides you with some background information on Yoga. First, I
give you a brief history of the discipline. Next, I explore the nature of stress and
the health benefits that are conferred as a result of regular Yoga practice. And
finally, I've included some practical tips for getting started and overcoming common stumbling blocks that may prevent you from committing to Yoga.

In Part Two, I delve into all the different techniques you can use to combat
stress. You'll find separate chapters on Yoga poses (*asanas*, or physical postures),
breathing practices (*pranayama*), and meditation. Because so many of us have

busy schedules, I've geared these exercises toward accessibility and ease of use. Most of the techniques in this book can be done anywhere, at any time, and for as little or as much time as you have available to you.

With *Big Yoga for Less Stress,* I've tried to give you a variety of options to help you manage and even eliminate stress. How you use this book is up to you. There's no right or wrong way to approach the material. Although I've provided some suggestions, there are no hard and fast rules about what you must do and when you should do it. The important thing is that you find a strategy that works for you, whether it's a quick five-minute meditation before work or a longer Yoga session that includes a movement sequence and some pranayama. Even the shortest practice can lift your mood and lower your stress levels. And the benefits are cumulative—the more regularly you're able to practice Yoga, the better you'll feel and the longer you'll feel better.

So don't wait! Make Big Yoga a part of your life today!

Part One

Yoga Basics

Before you embark on your journey to less stress, it's important that you learn a little bit about what you're getting into! Part One gives you a simple overview of Yoga: its history, its health benefits, and the information and equipment you will need to begin practicing this wonderful discipline. You'll also learn the basics of stress—where it comes from, how it works on the body, and what you can do to keep it from taking over your life.

In Chapter 1, you'll read about how Yoga evolved, moving out of India and into all the corners of the Earth. The teaching of Yoga has a long lineage that goes back thousands of years. At first, Yogic wisdom was transferred by oral tradition, handed down from teacher to student with no books or formal texts. In fact, the teachings had been around for hundreds of years before they were compiled and put on paper—well, actually, on palm leaves.

> "Regular practice of yoga can help you face the turmoil of life with steadiness and stability."
> —B.K.S. IYENGAR

In Chapter 2, I delve deep into the benefits of Yoga for stress relief. I discuss stress as a biological response and explain how scientists have viewed it over the years. You'll learn how stress is in fact responsible for many serious ailments. More important, I'll show you how Yoga has been shown to reduce and even eliminate stress.

In Chapter 3, I provide you with all the practical information you will need in order to get started in your Yoga practice. Although many of the techniques I discuss in Part Two require no extra equipment, I'll tell you about some props you may want to get to facilitate your moves. Later in the chapter, I offer tips on getting the most out of your practice.

Finally, Chapter 4 offers some advice on overcoming common stumbling blocks. Those of us who struggle to get through our crazy, hectic days know that there are many excuses that prevent us from practicing Yoga on a regular basis. Just remember: you don't have to do every pose every day, or sit for meditation twice a day. Even a little Yoga—be it five minutes of poses or five minutes of breath work—can give you significant stress relief. The important thing is that you incorporate Yoga into your life, making it a part of your daily routine, if possible.

Chapter 1

The Evolution of Yoga

The word *Yoga* comes from the Sanskrit root word *yug*, meaning to yoke or unite. Through the practice of exercise and breathing, Yoga unites our bodies, minds, and spirits, and brings us into a state of balance, making us feel still, renewed, and refreshed. Interestingly, the root word of *religion* has a similar meaning: to bind or connect. Although Yoga is not a religion, after practicing its exercises and breathing techniques, we connect to our higher selves. And when we come together to do Yoga, we receive the added benefit of connecting with each other and creating community.

Before you begin to learn about the practices of Yoga, let's take a minute to learn about where Yoga came from and how it became popular in the United States.

> "Yogas chitta vritti nirodhah
> Tada drastuh svarupe vasthanam
> *Yoga is the stilling of the thought waves in the mind*
> *Then the true self abides in its own nature.*"
> —PATANJALI, *YOGA SUTRAS*

THE ORIGINS OF YOGA

We don't know the exact origin of Yoga, but we do know that it emerged at least 5,000 years ago in the Indus Valley, an area that covered northern India and parts of neighboring Pakistan and Afghanistan. Yoga began as an inquiry into the nature of reality, asking the question, "Who am I?" Ancient Yogis developed various practices to help calm the mind and body, seeking to attain a state called *moksha*—pure, undifferentiated consciousness, a state of bliss. The ultimate purpose of Yoga is to become one with the divine within yourself.

As I mentioned earlier, although it is associated with many world religions, including Hinduism, Jainism, and Buddhism, Yoga is not itself a religious practice. Scholars tell us that, if anything, Yoga predates these faiths. In fact, some say that Yoga influenced and provided the philosophical underpinnings for much of Eastern religion. According to my teacher, Swami Satchidananda, Yoga is the "essence of all the religions."

Some of the first texts to incorporate Yogic philosophy were the Vedas, written between 1500 to 500 BCE. The four main books of the Vedas—the Rig-Veda, the Sama-Veda, the Yajur-Veda, and the Atharya-Veda—helped form the foundations of Indian culture and classical Hinduism. As the legend goes, the knowledge in these books was revealed to special poets or holy men called *rishis* by Brahma, the Universal Soul, God as Creator. Containing hymns, chants, prayers, liturgical formulas, and even magical spells, these texts were transmitted by word of mouth from teacher (*guru*) to student over hundreds of years. Much of what we know about Yoga today comes from the Vedas.

> "Ancient Vedic culture, which lays claim to being the first written spiritual tradition in the world, is much older than the loosely formed religion, Hinduism, that sprang from it. The spiritual practice of Yoga was part of Vedic culture long before Hinduism."
>
> —DEEPAK CHOPRA

Other important religious texts that integrates Yogic wisdom include the Bhagavad Gita, a sacred scripture that goes into detail on a number of concepts first laid out in the Upanishads (a special subsection of the Vedas), and the Yoga Sutras. The Yoga Sutras were compiled by the sage Patanjali, a man who is often referred to as the father of modern Yoga. It was written on palm leaves and contained 195 *sutras*—sutra meaning thread, as in the thread of an idea. These pithy sutras are the foundation of what is known today as Raja Yoga, a Yogic philosophy that incorporates practices from the eight separate but equal limbs on Patanjali's tree of Yoga, which you'll learn about on page 113. Today, the Yoga Sutras are still a primary text for Yoga professionals and spiritual seekers, who study its teachings to gain insight into the human psyche. Many modern Yoga masters, including my guru, have published special commentaries on the Yoga Sutras, helping to elaborate the meaning of the text's short, cryptic phrases for beginning students. You can find a few of my favorite commentaries by contemporary Yoga masters in the Resources section of this book.

By the time Patanjali compiled the Yoga Sutras, Yoga had already begun to spread from India to other parts of the Eastern world, influencing local religions and philosophy wherever it went. In turn, Yoga was also influenced by outside faiths and philosophies. Ideas were exchanged, and the practice of Yoga developed over time.

About Sanskrit

The Vedas, the Bhagavad Gita, and the Yoga Sutras were all written in Sanskrit, an ancient Indian language that was used in religious, philosophical, and literary texts. Today, Sanskrit is considered a "liturgical language"—that is, it's a language of worship, heard primarily in Hindu temples, and not a common tongue spoken at home. But Sanskrit also survives through the practice of Yoga; because many of the foundational texts for Yoga were written in this sacred language, most of the postures, meditations, and forms of breath work we use even now have Sanskrit names. Out of respect for this legacy, and because of the beneficial effect these words have on our consciousness, I've included the Sanskrit name for each exercise and its English equivalent whenever appropriate.

Politics and money have also had a hand in the evolution of Yoga. As Europe began to trade with Asia, Indian culture traveled west. In 1600, the East India Company—a conglomeration of British merchants—set out to trade with China and the Indian subcontinent, bringing back treasures such as cotton, silk, indigo dye, and tea to England. As Britain became increasingly dependent on these luxuries, the government stepped into India in order to protect its economic interests. What started out as a commercial venture became a national exercise in colonization. First unofficially through the East India Company, and then, beginning in 1857, through direct administration, India became a dominion of the British empire.

But cotton and silks weren't the only items of value to reach Britain from India—Yoga arrived, too! After claiming India for Britain in the nineteenth century, the British head of state, Queen Victoria, boldly took the title of Empress of India. Her interest in Indian things led to a fascination with Yoga, and Yogis were brought to court to perform for her amusement. Imagine the Queen watching a scantily

> *"Truth is one, paths are many."*
> —Mahatma Gandhi

clad Yogi walk over coals, stand on his head, or rest on a bed of nails. Today, these images seem like familiar caricatures, but in the prim-and-proper Victorian era, seeing a half-dressed man was shocking!

And so, although it was probably for all the wrong reasons, Yoga captured the imaginations of the rich and powerful. It was something new, interesting, and perhaps a little titillating, too. However, beyond the fascination with the Yogis' seemingly bizarre antics, there was a genuine interest in the way they had supreme control of their bodies. From then on, Yoga continued to grow and evolve.

EAST/WEST FUSION

After Yoga arrived in Europe, it eventually found its way to the United States near the end of the nineteenth century. In 1893, the eloquent Swami Vivekananda came to Chicago from India to speak about Hinduism at the Parliament of Religions, a conference held as part of the Columbian Exposition. This interfaith event marked the earliest formal gathering of representatives of Eastern and Western spiritual traditions from around the world. It was also the first opportunity Americans had to meet an authentic Yoga master and Hindu monk to discuss the lofty ideals of various religious traditions.

In 1920, another great Indian Yogi, Paramahansa Yogananda, came to America. Growing up in India under British rule, Yogananda gained a command of the English language as well as an affinity for the Western way of thinking. He traveled around the United States for the next thirty years, sharing his knowledge of Yoga and initiating followers into a meditation system called Kriya Yoga. Later in life, he was responsible for introducing Kriya Yoga to Mahatma Gandhi during a trip back home.

Yogananda had a love of chanting—one of the main practices of Bhakti Yoga, a branch of Yoga that emphasizes devotion as a way to liberate the mind from negativity. His *bhajans,* or devotional songs, are still sung all over the world today. Yogananda was very popular, partly due to his charming sweetness, childlike wonder at worldly matters, and ability to tell fascinating stories of the miracles that seemed to happen to and around him. His book, *Autobiography of a Yogi,* first published in 1946, remains one of the all-time bestsellers on the subject of Yoga; aspiring Yogis today find it a fascinating historical overview of the early days of Yoga in America.

OTHER DEVELOPMENTS IN HEALTH AND WELL-BEING

During the first decades of the twentieth century, other developments in health and well-being helped pave the way for larger-scale interest in Yoga. Increasingly, American thinkers saw a connection between mind and body, and subsequently began to develop programs to support and nurture both in natural, therapeutic ways. Many parallels can be seen between the discipline of Yoga and the practices set up by many of the American health innovators of the early 1900s.

Take, for instance, Dr. John H. Kellogg, the inventor of corn flakes. Kellogg's interest in health and natural cures inspired him not only to create breakfast cereals, but also to open the Battle Creek Sanitarium in Michigan in the early 1900s. This sanitarium prescribed many of the same things that were espoused in Yoga: sunbathing, vegetarian diet, exercise, and enemas. Kellogg, like the Yogis, believed the body was a living temple. He believed the colon was the source of most disease in the body, and that it should therefore be kept clean from above and below. These beliefs are strikingly similar to ancient Yogic texts on intestinal health.

Another early health entrepreneur, Paul Bragg, wrote a health column for the *Los Angeles Times* in the 1920s. The column expounded on his beliefs that deep breathing, fasting, juicing, and eating organic foods were the way to a long and healthy life. Many of these beliefs seem almost to have sprung from the deep well of Yogic wisdom. Bragg toured the country promoting his books, giving lectures and private consultations, and inspiring legions of followers, one of whom was the amazing fitness expert Jack LaLanne, who lived to the ripe old age of 97!

We can't be sure that any of these innovators were directly influenced by Yoga, but their popularity attests to the fact that Americans were ready to start thinking about their health and well-being in new and more holistic ways. People like Kellogg and Bragg set the stage for the growth of Yoga that would come in future decades.

WOODSTOCK RESURGENCE

After flourishing during the back-to-nature movement of the early twentieth century, interest in Yoga and health waned as Americans fought through the World Wars and the Depression. Yoga did not make a comeback until the 1960s and early 1970s, when a host of Indian Yoga masters came to America to lecture and demonstrate the Yogic lifestyle. Disgusted with the Vietnam War and the complicity of their parents' generation, young Americans were looking for a different way of thinking and living. Many of them found it in 1969 at Woodstock, one of the earliest and biggest celebrations of counterculture. There, they were introduced to Yoga through my teacher, Sri Swami Satchidananda, known by some as the "Woodstock Swami," because he was invited to open the event with simple peace chants, setting the tone for the entire weekend.

Swami Satchidananda had originally been invited to visit New York in 1966 by the artist Peter Max. Although he had only intended to stay for a few days, teaching Yoga to Peter and his friends, Swami Satchidananda found that Americans were very receptive to his thinking. What had started as a short visit became a life's work, bringing Integral Yoga to the United States and beyond.

Around the same time that Swami Satchidananda came to New York, his brother monk, Swami Vishnudevananda, came to Canada. This was no coincidence—both Yogis were students of Swami Sivananda, who, before his death in 1963, had urged them to bring Yoga to the West. It is purported that Swami Sivananda said to Swami Vishnudevananda, "People are waiting!" It was as if Swami Sivananda knew that Westerners were ready to learn the ancient wisdom of Yoga.

His Holiness
Sri Swami Satchidananda

The Reverend Sri Swami Satchidananda—known as Swamiji, and later, Gurudev—was born on December 22, 1914 in a small village in South India. Even as a child he had a pious nature, which was encouraged by his devout family. As a young adult, he worked in agriculture, mechanics, electronics, and cinematography. Later, he turned his attention to serious spiritual practice and studied with many great masters, including Sri Ramana Maharshi and Sri Aurobindo. When he met His Holiness Sri Swami Sivananda Saraswati of the Divine Life Society in Rishikesh, however, Swami Satchidananda knew that he had found his mentor and guru. He was initiated into the Paramahansa order of Sannyasa in 1949, and spent the rest of his life sharing his vast knowledge of Yoga and serving others—first in India, later in the United States, and ultimately all over the world.

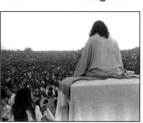

Swami Satchidananda
at Woodstock

In order to do this, Swami Satchidananda founded the Integral Yoga Institutes in 1966 to spread the ancient teachings of Yoga. While some Yoga schools primarily focus on the physical postures, Satchidananda's Integral Yoga takes a more expansive view of the practice, incorporating—or *integrating*—various types of Yoga. In addition to the physical postures of Hatha Yoga, Integral Yoga also involves pranayama, the breathing practices; Jnana Yoga, the yoga of self-reflection; Raja Yoga, the eight-fold path of liberation; Karma Yoga, the Yoga of action and selfless service; and Bhakti Yoga, the Yoga of devotion. For Satchidananda, a balanced practice that includes elements from each of these types of Yoga is the best way to achieve the final goal of moksha, or liberation—supreme happiness.

In 1980, Swamiji also created Yogaville, a spiritual community located in Buckingham, Virginia. Serving as the headquarters for Integral Yoga, the Yogaville community is built around the Satchidananda Ashram, a teaching center and retreat facility. Yogaville features five sacred sites, including the Light of Truth Universal Shrine (LOTUS), a temple that promotes interfaith dialogue and understanding. Yogaville is the culmination of Swami Satchidananda's vision for a "heaven on earth." It's a place where people of all backgrounds can come together to study and practice the principles of Integral Yoga.

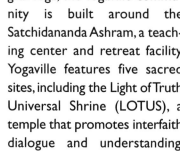

Swami Satchidananda took *mahasamadhi*—the soul's conscious exit from the body—on August 19, 2002 in South India. During his life, he was awarded the Martin Buber Award for Outstanding Service to Humanity, the Humanitarian Award of the B'nai Brith Anti-Defamation League, and the Albert Schweitzer Humanitarian Award. His body is interred at Yogaville in the Chidambaram Shrine, which is open to the public for prayer and meditation.

His Holiness
Swami Sivananda

Born Kuppuswami on September 8, 1887 in South India, Sivananda Saraswati was a vigorous and intelligent child. He attended medical school, and after graduation he worked as a doctor for ten years, often deferring fees for those who couldn't afford his care. In his late thirties, he began to feel a strong pull toward the renounced life and moved to Rishikesh, where he met his guru, Swami Vishwananda Saraswati. He was initiated into the Sannyasa order and given the name Sivananda. While continuing to help the sick, Swami Sivananda intensely practiced pranayama, meditation, and Hatha Yoga.

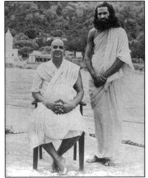

H.H. Sri Swami
Sivananda (seated)

Over time, Swami Sivananda developed his own style of Yoga, drawing on his medical expertise to create a hybrid form that emphasizes physical well-being and the avoidance of disease. Sivananda Yoga focuses on a particular sequence of asanas, or physical poses, that are said to be beneficial to all the organs and glands of the body. Breathing practices, deep relaxation, and meditation are also seen as critical to releasing stored-up toxins and harmonizing the systems of the body, helping you to live a more healthy life.

Swami Sivananda founded the Divine Life Society, an organization dedicated to spreading spiritual knowledge and teaching people about his style of Yoga. He also created the Sivananda Ayurvedic Pharmacy and organized the All-World Religions Federation. He wrote almost 300 books on various subjects—including metaphysics, religion, and spirituality—and trained many disciples who, in turn, became influential teachers of Yoga in their own rights. Swami Sivananda was devoted to the idea of the essential oneness of all religions, and his philosophy can be summed up in his famous sutra: *serve, love, give, purify, meditate, realize!*

Swami Vishnudevananda taught the Sivananda style of Yoga, first in Canada, and later in the United States. Other Yoga teachers who came to the West in the 1960s were Yogi Bhajan of the Kundalini Yoga tradition, Yogi Amrit Desai of the Kripalu Center, and Swami Muktananda of the Siddha Yoga tradition.

B.K.S. Iyengar, who recently left his body at the age of 95, is possibly the most renowned of all the contemporary Hatha Yoga masters. Though he rarely came to the United States, Iyengar is well known as an innovative teacher of teachers. His writings popularized the use of props and his adaptations of traditional asanas are used throughout the world. His style of Yoga continues to evolve today through the many books, CDs, and DVDs created by his students. Iyengar's teacher, Tirumalai Krishnamacharya, never came to the United States himself, but he also deserves a mention here. Considered by many to be the "Grandfather of Modern Yoga," Krishnamacharya taught many other famous contemporary Yoga students and teachers, including Indra Devi, Pattabhi Jois, and his own son, T.K.V. Desikachar.

Not to be forgotten are two important American teachers who helped spread and westernize Yoga, Lilias Folan and Richard Hittleman, who brought Yoga to television in the early 1970s. Other influential Yogis include Maharishi Mahesh Yogi, proponent of the Transcendental Meditation technique and the Beatles' guru; Ram Dass, the American who wrote the hippie bible *Be Here Now*; and founder of the Himalayan Institute, Swami Rama, who startled researchers in the 1970s with his ability to control his heart rate at will. Most of these pioneers of the western wave of Yoga are no longer with us, but their extensive contributions to the discipline remain. Contemporary Yoga owes them a huge debt of gratitude.

HATHA YOGA

Of the various types of Yoga currently practiced in the United States, Hatha Yoga is the most popular. The word *hatha* is combination of two ancient Sanskrit words—*ha*, meaning sun, and sometimes referred to as the warming or masculine side; and *tha*, meaning moon, sometimes referred to as the cooling, more receptive, feminine side. Thus *hatha* symbolically unites the right (masculine) and left (feminine) sides of the body, and merges energy patterns called *nadis* throughout the body. Hatha Yoga attempts to create a balance between mind, body, and these subtle energies. The practice of Hatha Yoga involves physical postures (asanas), breathing exercises (pranayamas), and cleansing practices (*kriyas*). Regular Hatha practice also focuses the mind, raises self-confidence, and improves mood. Over time, the physical postures will help you regulate your entire body, giving it strength, flexibility, and vitality. By preparing your body, you ready your mind for the higher consciousness known as samadhi—the most elevated state in Yoga.

Hatha Yoga is one of the many practices that make up Integral Yoga, and by extension, Big Yoga. The physical postures help to bring the body and mind into balance, and this balance is critical to leading a life free of stress. Because the Hatha poses can be challenging for some, I have adapted them so that everybody—and every body—can perform and benefit from them!

Chapter 2

How Yoga Can Help With Stress

Does your day look like this?

You sleep through your alarm because you were up late working on a project for work that was due yesterday. You rush to get the children up and dressed, then dash into the kitchen to put on the coffee, throw breakfast together for the family, and have a few bites of a stale bagel. You take a quick shower, get dressed, find out you're missing a button on the jacket you were going to wear, and have to reconfigure your outfit. Your daughter is having a meltdown because your dog has made a chew toy out of her favorite pair of shoes. Somehow, you get the children into the car and off to school, but then you realize you forgot to bring the flash drive containing the document you were working on last night, so you have to stop by the house again. Your partner is there, fuming because he spilled coffee on his dress shirt...

> *"Yoga has a sly, clever way of short-circuiting the mental patterns that cause anxiety."*
> —BAXTER BELL, YOGA EXPERT

Well, you get the idea.

Yoga has many benefits for your mind and your body. But it has one benefit that deserves special mention—and chances are, if you've picked up this book, you already know what that benefit is. With its emphasis on uniting the body, mind, and spirit, Yoga is fantastic for relieving stress.

In this chapter, I'll explain what stress is and why Yoga is such a powerful tool for managing it. Although the types of stress we experience today are very different from those experienced by ancient Yogis, the techniques developed by these spiritual gurus can help you bring balance and calm back into your life. What's more, the healing powers of Yoga will improve other aspects of your health and wellbeing. Try Yoga, and feel a difference today!

WHAT IS STRESS?

Stress is a natural evolutionary response that developed in order to help ancient humans deal with life-threatening situations—an attack by a hungry tiger, for example. Confronted by that hungry tiger, ancient humans had a choice: fight or flight. That is, they could either defend themselves against the attack (fight), or they could escape (flight). Over time, the human body evolved to facilitate both responses. In the face of danger, your body releases special hormones that enable you to react rapidly and expediently. As a result, your breathing increases and your heart rate accelerates, helping pump blood faster through your body to provide oxygen to your muscles so you can move more quickly and easily. Your digestion rate slows or stops, allowing more of your energy to be devoted toward fight or flight. And you develop a kind of tunnel vision, a narrowing of your peripheral vision that enables you to focus solely on the source of the danger. These are just some of the changes your body goes through as part of the stress response.

For ancient humans, the stress response was a good thing. It helped them to survive in scenarios in which they might ordinarily have died. In ancient times, as soon as the threat was eliminated (that is, the hungry tiger was either killed or left far behind), the stress response ended, and the body went back to its normal, balanced state. Today, the situation is much different. While most of us don't spend our days combating tigers, we now have to deal with many sources of lower-grade stress on a regular basis. Unfortunately, your body doesn't care whether you're fighting off tigers or trying to meet a deadline at work; your stress response is the same. The same hormones flood your body, and the same physical changes occur. Worse still, it's often difficult or even impossible to eliminate the sources of modern stress, so your body continues to churn out hormones as you continue to try to cope.

As Hungarian endocrinologist Hans Selye showed in the 1930s, the results of this chronic stress—a collection of physiological responses he called *General Adaptation Syndrome*—can be deeply harmful to your body. Considered the father of modern stress research, Selye introduced the idea that chronic stress contributes to the development of serious medical problems. As the body becomes exhausted by its attempts to deal with chronic stress, it loses its ability to function normally and can't return to a balanced state, leaving the door open to disease and illness. Advances in stress research continue today, aided by our ever-expanding knowledge of biochemistry and physiology.

GOOD STRESS VERSUS BAD STRESS

As you saw earlier, not all stress is bad. Some types of stress help us achieve goals and improve our lives. Hans Selye used the term *eustress* to describe this "positive," or useful, stress. As long as the stress is manageable, limited in duration, and directed toward a greater good, you can actually benefit from it.

Exercise is a great example of positive stress. When you stress your muscles during a short workout—putting them under strain and forcing them to work hard—you become stronger and more fit. Work out for too long, however, and your good stress turns to bad stress; you receive diminishing returns from your exercise and put yourself at risk for injury. The key is to find the right amount of stress. According to researcher Bruce McEwen, there are three different types of stress: *positive stress, tolerable stress,* and *toxic stress. Positive stress* is good stress, the kind that allows you to not only meet challenges, but to thrive and prosper as a result of your successful efforts. For example, positive stress occurs when you're taking a test for which you've adequately prepared: the stress helps keep you alert and focused so that you can ace the exam. It's a short-term form of stress—once the test is over, after an hour or so, the stress evaporates.

Tolerable stress occurs when you encounter challenges or ongoing conflicts that are difficult to deal with, but not unmanageable. In other words, you can *tolerate* the stress, often with the help of supportive friends or family members. Like positive stress, tolerable stress occurs over a fairly limited period of time, though it's usually longer in duration than the situations in which positive stress occurs. For example, if somebody breaks into your house and steals your computer and personal documents and jewelry, you may have a hard time replacing or compensating for the loss of these valuables and feeling safe in your home again. But with the support and assistance of your friends or spouse or children, you will eventually feel better.

> "Episodic stress is a gift to help us deal with life, but chronic stress diverts energy from digestion and the reproductive organs, creating long-term wasting diseases."
> —SWAMI VIDYANANDA MA, SENIOR MONK AT THE SATCHIDANANDA ASHRAM

If you lack that soothing support network, however, tolerable stress can very quickly turn into *toxic stress.* As the name implies, toxic stress is the kind of stress that can seriously damage your health and wellness. It is intense—often more so than in tolerable stress—prolonged, and cannot be buffered by friends or family. Examples of toxic stress include situations of poverty or ongoing verbal or physical abuse, but can be less extreme, too. Everybody reacts to stress differently; for some, stressors that might ordinarily be tolerable (unemployment, death in the family, etc.) may accumulate over time, resulting in toxic stress. One person's tolerable stress is another person's toxic stress. People who already suffer from low self-esteem, anxiety, or depression may feel unable to handle situations that more confident people find manageable.

Toxic stress is no joke. As you'll see, the effects of toxic stress can be quite dramatic.

THE EFFECTS OF CHRONIC STRESS

Although each of us reacts differently to stress, most of us know how it feels. Personally, I get butterflies in my stomach, my heart starts to race, and my neck tightens. Maybe you get sweaty palms, chest pains, or a blinding headache. And perhaps another person feels lightheaded or sick to her stomach.

As I explained earlier, all of these physical changes occur as part of your body's evolutionary and automatic "fight or flight" response. The changes enable you to focus on and neutralize the stressful situation, either by fighting it or fleeing it. Your muscles tense up, readying themselves for action. Your heart beats faster to get more blood and oxygen to your muscles and your blood's clotting ability is enhanced—a carryover from ancient times, when having improved clotting ability meant that if you were attacked by a tiger, you wouldn't bleed to death as quickly. Your digestion shuts down so that your body can devote more attention to dealing with the stressor; at the same time, your metabolism speeds up, encouraging your body to burn fat and so that you have more energy immediately available.

Most of the time, these sensations go away fairly quickly as we deal with the stressful situation at hand. But what happens to your body when you're exposed to chronic, toxic stress? All those changes persist. Your blood pressure remains high and your heart continues to beat quickly, your muscles stay tense, and your digestion may be impaired. Scientists have found that there are many more serious and long-term health problems that develop as a result of chronic stress. Recent studies have indicated that chronic stress can cause systemic inflammation; in turn, that inflammation can destroy brain cells. As a result, McEwen says, chronic stress can aggravate or increase the risk of heart disease, depression, diabetes, Alzheimer's disease, arthritis, and even cancer. Others have linked chronic stress to obesity, diabetes, reproductive problems, gastrointestinal disorders, and drug or alcohol abuse.

Chronic stress may also harm your body on a genetic level. Dr. Dean Ornish, a researcher best known for his holistic approach to treating and reversing heart disease, has done extensive work into the effects of stress on health and wellness. Ornish and others found that chronic stress damages telomeres, the little protective caps at the end of chromosomes, the structures that contain our DNA. Telomeres are often compared to the plastic coverings at the end of shoelaces; they prevent the contents of the chromosomes from unraveling or being lost during the cell replication process. Telomeres naturally shorten as they age; in fact, they're usually considered to be markers of the aging process. Unfortunately, other factors—including stress—can hasten their shortening. This is a problem, scientists say, because short telomeres can prevent your cells from replicating properly. Instead of healthy cells, dead or faulty cells are produced, making it difficult for your body to function normally. Shorter telomeres have been linked to many age-related diseases, including osteoporosis, dementia, obesity, diabetes, heart disease, and certain kinds of cancer.

But Dr. Ornish has good news: telomere shrinkage is reversible! By making a number of simple lifestyle changes, you can actually lengthen your telomeres, thus reducing your risk of the age-related diseases mentioned earlier. Like me, Ornish was a student of Sri Swami Satchidananda. As a result, many of the lifestyle changes he advocates—including a vegetarian diet and light exercise—are based on Satchidananda's teachings. Most important, Ornish recommends adopting a program of stress management that includes Yoga and meditation. In a 2009 study undertaken by Ornish and his colleagues at UCLA, patients who made these lifestyle changes saw a significant increase in their telomere length. Certain disease-preventing genes were turned on, while other disease-promoting genes were turned off.

Many other scientists have investigated the ways by which stress management helps ward off disease and decline. Another medical pioneer in the field of stress management is Dr. Herbert Benson, a cardiologist who teaches at Harvard Medical School and the founder of the Benson-Henry Institute for Mind Body medicine. As a cardiologist, Dr. Benson was initially intrigued by the ways that stress affects blood pressure and other heart problems. Over time, he has dedicated his career to researching the many different ways in which stress affects human health. According to Dr. Benson, between 60 and 90 percent of all visits to the doctor are for conditions related to stress—that's a lot of pain and discomfort that could potentially be avoided! Moreover, Dr. Benson found that Yoga, meditation, and other relaxation techniques seemed to stimulate certain disease-fighting genes that were not active in people who didn't practice relaxation.

Like Dr. Ornish, Dr. Benson believes in the importance of taking a holistic approach to health. For Benson, mind and body are intimately linked. Accordingly, Benson proposes that the best representation of good healthcare is a three-legged stool, in which pharmaceuticals, surgeries and other procedures, and self-care each play equally important roles.

At the beginning of his career, Benson paid particular attention to meditation. Meditation, Benson found, triggers a "relaxation response" that counteracts the stress response. Instead of "fight or flight," meditation teaches us to "rest and digest." Benson's early studies showed that patients who practiced Transcendental Meditation experienced lower heart rates, a decrease in metabolism and muscle tension, slower breathing, and slower brainwaves. Later, Benson broadened his scope; subsequent studies showed that other techniques—including stretching, progressive muscle relaxation, diaphragmatic breathing, guided imagery, and even prayer—achieved effects similar to Transcendental Meditation. I'll touch on these techniques in later chapters.

Clearly, Yoga and meditation are not merely luxuries to be indulged in when we have the time. As Benson and Ornish have shown us, these stress management techniques are in fact essential if you want to avoid and even reverse certain kinds of disease. Indeed, studies have shown us again and again that we can live better and longer just by adopting a few simple lifestyle changes. Let's now take a look at how conscious self-care can improve your life.

THE BENEFITS OF YOGA

Today, Yoga is a booming American business. There are over 20.4 million people practicing Yoga in this country alone. And those 20.4 million people have spent $10.3 billion a year on Yoga classes, Yoga DVDs, Yoga equipment, Yoga clothing, Yoga retreats, and Yoga magazines.

"Yoga teaches us to cure what need not be endured and endure what cannot be cured"
—B.K.S. IYENGAR

Yoga has become ubiquitous in the United States—and for good reason. While traditional exercises are excellent for strengthening your body, Yoga works your body, mind, *and* spirit, creating harmony between them. As a result, its effects are more powerful and far-reaching. Below, you'll learn how Yoga provides many benefits to those of us who decide to use it as a tool for stress management.

Improves Overall Fitness

If you've been struggling with stress, you may have given up on exercise. With so many other things to do, many of us find we just don't have the time to devote to a workout. Once we fall off the exercise wagon, it's difficult to get back on. You may dread going back to the gym because you feel out of shape and out of place. I know from my own personal struggles with weight, impulse control, and dietary indiscretions that I can slip into a downward spiral when I don't feel like exercising. Once I stop moving my body, it starts to rebel. I think to myself, "Oh, my hips are a little achy," or "Gee, my face looks puffy," and later, "Ouch! My back is killing me!" Pretty soon, all I want to do is sit on the couch and stare into space. So believe me, I've been there!

If you're out of shape, Yoga is a great way to improve your general fitness.

The obvious benefit is that you will gain flexibility. As you perform the Yoga stretches found in Part Two of this book, you'll notice your muscles and joints loosening up. You'll feel lighter and less achy—and as you increase your mobility, you'll realize you suddenly feel more like being active. In addition, if you take part in other forms of vigorous exercise, the flexibility you gain from Yoga will help protect you against injury and allow you to feel more at home in your body.

You may be surprised to learn that Yoga also improves your muscular strength and endurance. Your bones will become stronger and you'll develop better balance, too! Don't worry about not being able to perform all the exercises perfectly. The poses and stretches in this book are simple, making it easy for you to be successful in your workout.

Cleans Out Toxins

When we're stressed, sometimes we stop taking good care of ourselves. We eat poorly, we don't exercise, and we don't get as much sleep as we'd like. As a result, toxins build up in our bodies, making us feel bloated and tired. Ordinarily, these harmful substances would be flushed out by your lymph system, a part of your immune system that is often referred to as the body's sewers. But because your lymph system moves more slowly when you're less active, and because it has to deal with a higher volume of toxins due to your poor eating and sleeping habits, your lymph system quickly becomes overwhelmed, and circulates less efficiently than usual.

Yoga can help get your lymph moving again! As you shift in and out of the Yoga postures, contracting and relaxing muscles, you exert gentle pressure on your tissues and internal organs. This pressure helps to propel the lymph so that it can remove toxins and fight infections.

Improves Mood

Yoga has been shown to alleviate depression and anxiety, two byproducts of stress. Studies show that Yoga actually increases brain levels of neurotransmitters like GABA, serotonin, and dopamine—special chemicals that help you feel happier and more relaxed. But you don't need science to realize that the mood-enhancing effect of Yoga is real. As you tune into your body during Yoga, you shift your attention away from the sources of your sadness or worry, focusing instead on your physical sensations: the sound of your breath as you move, the gentle rising and falling of your abdomen, the way your muscles feel as you tense and relax them. This shift in perspective allows you to see the bigger picture and feel at peace with the world.

Facilitates Sleep

Is there anything better than a good night's sleep to help soothe the worries of the day? Unfortunately, when you're stressed out, you're much more likely to have insomnia or other sleep problems. If you've been having trouble falling or staying asleep, Yoga can help. Researchers at Harvard Medical School found that people who practiced Yoga every day for eight weeks saw improvements in sleep efficiency (the amount of time actually spent sleeping while in bed), total sleep time, total wake time, and the amount of time it took to fall asleep.

Another study suggested that Yoga and meditation were effective in encouraging sleep because these practices stimulate the production of melatonin, a hormone that helps regulate your circadian rhythms—among them, the "sleep-wake" cycle. Melatonin can also promote a feeling of well-being, helping to alleviate any anxieties that prevent you from getting a good night's rest. This probably makes intuitive sense to you: when you sleep better, your mood also improves, and you're less cranky during the day. What's more, with the proper amount of sleep, your risk for certain medical conditions—including heart disease—is also reduced.

Deep breathing, chanting, and guided progressive relaxation are just some of the ways you can bring your mind into stillness, so that when your head hits the pillow, you can sleep like a baby, allowing your body to restore itself. When we practice these Yoga techniques, we also become experts in controlling the stress response, enabling us to not only remove one obstacle to sleep, but also maintain vitality and prevent disease.

Strengthens the Immune System

You have already learned how chronic stress impairs your immune system, making you susceptible to illness. Regular meditation has been shown to boost the immune system. And the effects are lasting—studies show that even if you stop meditating, the benefits continue for weeks afterwards. Yoga helps by reducing your blood levels of cortisol, the stress hormone, which seems to interfere with the effectiveness of white blood cells, your body's first responders to germs and other disease-carrying agents. Moreover, as you read earlier, Yoga gets your lymph circulating, helping your body get rid of toxins and waste. A recent study has also suggested that Yoga may improve immunity on a genetic level, permanently "turning on" specific genes that help stimulate and maintain the immune system.

Helps Manage or Reverse Serious Health Conditions

As you read earlier, chronic stress is a risk factor for many medical problems and diseases. Because Yoga is so good at reducing stress and strengthening your immune system, it can be very useful for managing or even reversing serious health conditions. Scientists like Dr. Ornish and Dr. Benson have devoted a lot of research to demonstrating Yoga's positive effects on disease. Yoga is great for people who are at risk for heart disease, helping to lower heart rate and blood pressure. It has also been shown to lower levels of total cholesterol, LDL ("bad") cholesterol, and triglycerides—further reducing the risk of heart disease, metabolic syndrome, diabetes, and overweight/obesity. There is even some evidence that Yoga helps balance blood sugar. One recent study indicated that patients with type 2 diabetes were able to reduce their need for oral medications after practicing Yoga regularly.

Research shows that Yoga decreases pain and increases mobility in people who suffer from chronic lower-back pain. And, as I mentioned earlier, Yoga can help relieve anxiety, depression, and insomnia. Because some poses expand the chest, some studies show that Yoga can be beneficial for the treatment of asthma and emphysema. Other research even indicates that regular Yoga practice alleviates pain from arthritis and other inflammatory conditions. In addition, the movements involved in Yoga massage your internal organs, helping to promote good bowel health and digestion.

YOGA HEALS

By this point, you should have an appreciation for how deeply stress affects all of us. You should also have a good understanding of Yoga's profound capacity not only to relieve stress, but to reduce or even eliminate many health problems associated with stress. Studies show that Yoga actually has healing powers!

But you don't have to be unwell to take advantage of those healing powers. Regular Yoga practice more generally helps keep your body in good condition. After you start doing Yoga, you'll notice that you start to feel better, both physically and mentally. Yoga is a wonderful tonic for all that ails you—the daily grind, your aches and pains, your emotional fatigue. Yoga makes your mind sharp and your mood positive. You may even find you are experiencing a deeper spiritual connection with yourself and the world.

Make Yoga a central part of your stress management plan, and prepare to reap the benefits!

Chapter 3

Beginning Your Yoga Practice

Now that you know a bit about how Yoga can help you reduce stress, you are probably excited to get started. I've designed this book to make it easier than ever before to work Yoga poses, breathing practices, and meditation into your busy day. Most of the techniques I discuss in Part Two require no special equipment whatsoever. Many of these exercises can be done anywhere, and at any time. That way, you never have to skip out on a stress management session.

> "Yoga is not about touching your toes. It's about unlocking your ideas about what you want, where you think you can go, and what you will achieve when you get there."
> —CYNDI LEE, YOGA EXPERT

Before you flip through to Part Two, however, there are a few practical matters you will want to consider. In this chapter, I'll explain some precautions and share tips on how to get the most out of your sessions. Yoga should help relieve stress—not cause it!

COMMON YOGA EQUIPMENT

With every form of exercise, it's best to have the right equipment and wear appropriate clothing. Yoga is no exception. The nice thing about Yoga, though, is that you don't have to empty your bank account in order to do it right. And, as I mentioned earlier, many of the exercises and techniques in this book call for nothing more than a chair and a little free time. You don't need to buy anything—you probably have everything you need already!

Still, there are a number of props that can help make your practice a little easier, especially if you are thinking about getting into Yoga on a more intensive basis. Let's look at some of the items you might want to have handy.

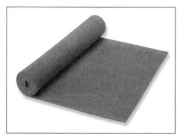

A Mat

You will want to perform your Yoga poses on some type of mat. These days, Yoga is most often done on mats made of rubber or PVC. These mats are sticky, making it easier for feet to adhere to them in the standing poses. They can be bought online, at department stores, or at sporting good stores. And they can be doubled up if you need extra cushioning under your knees or buttocks. If you don't want to buy a mat, feel free to use a beach towel you might have lying around the house; it will work just fine.

A Chair

You'll need a chair for two of the sequences in this book. The chair should be sturdy, with a straight back. The seat can be cushioned for greater comfort. It's also helpful to keep a chair handy if you're doing exercises on the floor, in case you need help getting up.

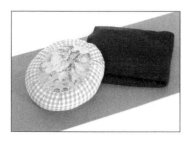

A Blanket or Pillow

For seated exercises and meditations, it can be more comfortable to sit on a folded blanket or pillow. The folded blanket raises your buttocks, allowing your knees to relax and drop toward the floor. It also helps release tension in your groin. Again, you can use something you already have at home, or you can order a fancy blanket or pillow online.

Traditional Japanese meditation pillows—sometimes referred to as a *zafus*—are usually round and have a strap for easy carrying. There are also newer types of meditation pillows that are crescent-shaped or rectangular. Moreover, pillows come in all different sizes; you should pick the one that feels right to you. But don't forget, you also have pillows right there on your couch that might do the trick.

A Sweater

At the end of my classes, I talk students through a deep relaxation that lasts anywhere from five to fifteen minutes. I recommend they bring a sweater to put on before we start so they don't get chilled. You might want to do the same. Or use a shawl—a large, soft pashmina works great and makes you feel pampered, too!

An Outfit

Yoga clothing should be comfortable. Period. It shouldn't constrict you in any way or bind you at the waist. A stretch-waisted pant and a loose top are ideal, though some people feel most comfortable in a hoodie and sweats. These days a variety of Yoga clothes are available online and from many big-box chains in sizes up to 3X and 4X. Personally, I like a little support in my Yoga duds, and usually wear something that is mostly cotton with some Lycra in it.

Mala Beads

You might also consider having some mala beads on hand for your meditation sessions. Mala beads are prayer necklaces made of 108 beads plus a center bead, or *mehru.* They can be made of many different materials—from humble sandlewood to precious stones like citrine, amethyst, and crystal. Originally from the Middle East, mala beads were brought west after European crusaders observed Muslims praying with them. In the west, these mala beads evolved into the rosary. The reason prayer beads and rosaries are used in so many diverse traditions is because they effectively help keep the mind focused on a prayer or mantra. After each mantra repetition, for instance, "All is one," or "om 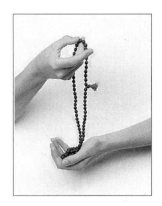 shanti" (see page 142), you move on to the next bead until you come to the *mehru.* Then, simply turn the beads around and continue for as long as you like.

TIPS FOR GETTING THE MOST OUT OF YOUR YOGA PRACTICE

In addition to gathering or purchasing props, there are a number of things you can do to prepare for Yoga so that you get the most out of your practice. We all lead hectic, demanding lives, and Yoga can help us put everything in perspective. Here are some ways to maximize the benefits of your Yoga sessions.

Practice on an Empty Stomach

Wait at least two to four hours after your last big meal, and an hour or longer after a snack, before practicing Yoga. An empty stomach is preferred here because you want your body to assimilate all the benefits of your practice and not have energy drained away by the process of digestion. Also, you will be more comfortable exercising without a full stomach, which can cause or aggravate a hiatal hernia.

After your Yoga session, have a glass of water. This water will help flush out any toxins that were released through your practice, and will help bring you out of Yoga mode and back into daily life.

Shower

Come to your practice clean and empty. Yoga is a sacred practice, and you should clean yourself up before participating, just as you would before church or temple. Try to have your morning elimination and shower before you begin. If you practice in the evening, a comfortable change of clothes and a quick wash of your face and hands should suffice. In addition, your Yoga practice will cause you to sweat a little and eliminate toxins, so it's better to start out fresh.

Remove Obstacles to Movement

If you wear a watch, large earrings, necklaces, or any other jewelry, you may want to remove them before you begin so they do not get in your way. Also, if you have long hair, you will probably want to tie it back.

Have a Special Yoga Mat

When you use the same mat or towel over and over, it begins to feel familiar. It's easy to settle down there, because you have settled down there before. You can feel that you are at home on your mat, even when you're in a Yoga studio with twenty other students. Because you're accustomed to using your special mat or towel, you have fewer distractions to prevent you from getting the most out of your practice.

Create a Dedicated Yoga Space

While you can do Yoga anywhere, I encourage you to create a niche in your home that will serve as a sort of an altar. At the very least, have a special candle that you only light during meditation and the Yoga poses. The candle will help you remember that you are light.

In addition to the candle, you may also want to keep an image of a saintly person in your special Yoga space. For instance, when my children were little, I kept a picture of Mother Mary on my altar to inspire me to be a good mother. Other times, I used a picture of my own mother, who also inspired me. A friend of mine keeps a picture of Oprah on her altar! If you want something religious, your neighborhood Yoga studio or New Age bookstore will have pictures, statues, and religious art from a wide variety of faiths, so go check them out and find one that speaks to you. Lord Buddha once said, "As we think, so we become." By meditating on a person who inspires you, you may begin to take on some of his or her supreme qualities.

I like to bring flowers to the altar to show my respect. Another nice accessory for your altar is a concentric geometric pattern called a *mandala* or *yantra. Mandala* is a combination of two ancient Sanskrit words meaning "having" and "essence." Mandalas and yantras are visual representations of a sacred sound, such as "om," or symbolic depictions of the cosmos themselves. In the center of the diagram there is often a red dot called a *bindu,* and by gazing at it, you may experience the holy vibration of that sound at a very subtle level. You may even experience a feeling of oneness with the entire cosmos! For more information, see the inset on page 124.

Set the Mood

If you're practicing in the privacy of your own home, light a candle, display some flowers, or put on some soft music to set a peaceful, relaxing mood. Incense can help contribute to this mood; light it fifteen minutes before you begin so the air isn't too smoky. Make sure any music you play is kept at a low volume, so that

Sitting Comfortably for Your Practice

For the breathing practices and for meditation, I recommend sitting on the floor in an easy cross-legged position known as *sukhasana,* as long as it's comfortable or you (see page 95). Use a pillow or folded blanket under your buttocks to raise it up so that your knees relax down toward the floor. You can also add pillows under each knee to avoid any strain. Comfort is the goal here. If this position isn't comfortable, try extending your legs out in front, and perhaps sit with your back against a wall for support.

Another option is to sit on a chair. For breath work, it's best to sit forward in the chair, with your feet flat on the floor or resting on a bolster or pillow. You want to be steady. For meditation, sit back in the chair, using the back of the chair for support. Again, your feet should be resting either on the floor (if you have long legs) or on a pillow or bolster placed on the floor (if your feet don't reach the ground while sitting back in the chair).

What about lying down for meditation? Unless you're getting ready for bed, I don't recommend it. It can be helpful to lie in bed for meditation as a preface to a good night's sleep, but you'll never get out of bed if you do it in the morning!

it will not distract you and draw your awareness away from your practice. If you're doing Yoga at the office, begin with a short affirmation or prayer. This allows you to consciously move your awareness out of work mode and into Yoga mode. You can also end your practice with a blessing or the same affirmation or prayer to help you move back into work mode.

Get Fresh Air

The room in which you practice Yoga should be warm and comfortable. But if it's not too cold or windy outside, open a window to let in some fresh air. If you want to practice outside instead, that's great, but avoid doing so in direct sunlight during the heat of the day.

Minimize Distractions

Keep your awareness within. If you're practicing at home, put away your cell phone. Turn down the volume on your home phone so you aren't listening to it ring and won't pay attention to the answering machine as it's picking up your messages. If you're practicing in a Yoga studio, try not to compare yourself to anyone in the room—not even yourself. Yoga is not a competitive sport; rather, it's a method of transformation. If you try to match the expertise of your teacher or a fellow student, you may hurt yourself. The best way to avoid injury is to honor your body and pay attention to what you're feeling. Your ability to observe your body will be enhanced over time, and you'll find yourself bringing consciousness to every part of your body.

Keep Your Breath Full and Relaxed

Yogic breathing brings energy to every part of the body. As you'll learn in Chapter 6, when there's more breath, there's more oxygen; more oxygen brings more *prana*, and more prana brings more joy and more vitality. That's what it's all about! In Yoga, you always breathe through your nose, with your mouth closed, unless otherwise indicated. The breath, though deep, is relaxed—there should never be a sound of gasping or grunting—and is almost never held during the asana practice.

Don't Use a Mirror

Do not scrutinize your every move in front of a mirror—at least not right away. It's important that you develop an internal consciousness of your body, knowing what you feel like on the inside without getting hung up on what you look like on the outside. As you practice, bring your awareness within, focusing on how you feel. When you become more familiar with the poses, you can check your alignment in a mirror, especially if you are doing Yoga at home without an instructor.

Shorten Your Practice if You're Pressured for Time

Your Yoga practice is flexible—you can do as much or as little as you can fit into your schedule. You don't have to do an entire movement sequence every day. If you only have time for one or two poses, that's fine; try to add in a brief relaxation and some deep breathing. Many people find that just doing a short meditation is helpful. Feel free to mix it up, and do what you can to get in a session daily. That way, you'll be able to maintain a consistent practice.

SOME WORDS OF CAUTION

The primary precaution I offer beginning Yoga students is to take it easy. We Westerners are highly competitive, so it's not unusual for new students to overdo it in an effort to "get it right," to show off a little, or to look like the models in the pictures. Trust me—it's not worth it. Respect your body at all times. Yoga is not a sport in which you should be trying to outdo your opponent or yourself. For instance, you may find you're more flexible on one side than the other, or that today you can't stretch as far in a pose as you could yesterday. This is not unusual. It's fine to make these observations, but in Yoga we learn not to judge ourselves or find ourselves lacking.

If you have health issues such as high blood pressure or arthritis, any physical limitations because of your weight, or any lack of flexibility because of your age, please check with a trusted medical professional before beginning Yoga. With practice and dedication, you may find that you begin to recover from your ailments.

My teacher, Sri Swami Satchidananda, always said, "Health is your birthright!" Your beautiful body is designed to move, and Yoga practice will help you either maintain or regain an ease of movement, giving you a spring in your step, a smile on your face, and a twinkle in your eye. Soon, simple everyday chores that may be difficult for you now—like making the bed or getting in and out of the car—will become effortless.

YOGIC DIET

Once you have made the decision to purify your system with Yoga, you might want to take some time to analyze your diet. The foods you eat can make an enormous difference to your mood and state of mind. Choose foods that make you healthy and calm. Become more aware about what you put into your body, and eat life-giving foods—essentially, more veggies and less junk. Get local, organic produce whenever possible, and live by the simple idea of "whole foods, eaten whole."

The Yogic diet recommended by my teacher, Swami Satchidananda, was strictly vegetarian. Because it causes no harm to any sentient being, a vegetarian diet puts you in alignment with a concept from the first limb of the tree of Yoga: the idea of *ahimsa,* or nonviolence (see page 132). My teacher, Swamiji, would give the example of animals in the zoo. The carnivores (meat-eaters), such as lions and tigers, are restless, pacing their cages. By contrast, the animals that are herbivores (plant-eaters), including the elephants, horses, and cows, are peaceful, but certainly not lacking in strength.

Swamiji also pointed out that the anatomy of herbivores is different from that of carnivores. Lions and tigers have big, sharp teeth made for tearing meat from the bone, and short digestive tracts to get the digested food out of the system. Have you ever given a hungry dog a bite of meat? He doesn't even chew it; he just gobbles it down! By comparison, goats, cows, and other grazing animals have flatter teeth made for chewing. And they have much longer digestive tracts— like ours. Human intestines can be nearly thirty feet long! Grains take longer to break down than meat, and our longer digestive tracts enable our bodies to extract all the nutrients out of them.

Science backs the adoption of a vegetarian diet. As stress expert and Yoga enthusiast Dr. Dean Ornish has shown us, a vegetarian diet can help treat and even reverse heart disease. Vegetarian diets have also been demonstrated to lower the risk of certain types of cancer, diabetes, obesity, and hypertension (high blood pressure).

That said, a vegetarian diet is certainly not a requirement for Yoga, or for stress relief! Omnivores will still get great results from the exercises and techniques discussed in this book. My point is merely that a vegetarian diet may help you achieve better health and higher levels of success in your practice of Yoga. The main thing, however, is that you try to incorporate some aspects of the Yogic lifestyle into your own life. Whatever you can do—be it a vegetarian diet, a few minutes of meditation, some breath work, or a brief routine of Yoga movements—will contribute to your sense of calm and well-being.

Chapter 4

Overcoming stumbling Blocks

If done regularly, Yoga can have many benefits for the body and mind. The problem is, when you're busy and stressed out, daily practice can seem impossible. But it's a good idea to do Yoga as often as you can. Regularity is the key to getting the results you're looking for, and you're worth it! Try to set aside time every day to do a little stretching and breathing. You'll be pleasantly surprised to see how quickly your body responds. Nike got it right—you need to "just do it!"

> *"Motivation is what gets you started. Habit is what keeps you going."*
> —JIM RYUN,
> ATHLETE AND POLITICIAN

Too often, excuses get in the way. We all have our own reasons for not getting on the Yoga mat on any given day. I've been practicing Yoga for over thirty years and I still have an encyclopedia full of excuses! To overcome these excuses, some days, I simply act as if I want to do my exercises. Acting "as if" is a very useful tool in making positive changes in our lives. William James, the father of American psychology, was credited with coming up with the idea. He claimed, "If you want a quality, act as if you already had it." When you pretend you want to do something, a part of your brain directs your behavior and outlook to corrrespond to the action you pretend to want. When I need to do my Yoga even though I'm not feeling it, I'll do something that gets me closer to actually practicing, like putting on my sweatpants or sitting on my meditation pillow. From there, I find myself moving to my mat, and once I'm on the mat, I fall into a comforting routine and am glad I did.

This chapter discusses various common excuses people use to avoid Yoga, and offers some tricks to help you transcend them.

I DON'T HAVE ENOUGH TIME

I think we've all had this excuse at one point or another. Our culture has scheduled itself into oblivion. We are constantly trying to beat the clock, and are beating ourselves up in the process! If like most people these days, you are trying to juggle a career, a family, community sevice, exercise, and aspirations for a spiritual life, you may find your needs are at the bottom of the deck.

The next time you are feeling overwhelmed and pressured for time, remind yourself that you still can, and should, squeeze in some Yoga. Do a little breathwork, or meditate. If you choose to do some Yoga movements, remember that you don't have to do every pose every time in order to make your routine count. In fact, it's much better to do a simple, short practice regularly than it is to do a long, intense practice once or twice a month. You also may find you prefer certain poses more than others. That's fine. All that means is that your inner guru, or teacher, is helping you discover what you need.

> *"Life moves pretty fast. If you don't stop and look around once in a while, you could miss it."*
> —FERRIS BUELLER'S DAY OFF

I know it sounds a little farfetched, but regular Yoga practice can actually make time seem to expand by improving your physical and mental capabilities and awareness. Solutions to problems will become more obvious, and the length of time it takes you to perform various activities will be reduced. In short, Yoga can make you feel like you have more time.

I DON'T HAVE A PLACE TO DO YOGA

Many people say they don't have a proper space in which to practice yoga. For the purposes of this book, this ought to be a nonissue! The great thing about the exercises and techniques in this book is that they can be completed anywhere and at any time. Strictly speaking, you don't *need* to have a special sanctuary in which to meditate or do breath work.

At the same time, it's true that you can elevate your Yoga practice by performing it in a sacred space. As I discussed in the previous chapter, it can be useful to create a special area in your home, in which you keep candles, religious or inspiring images, and your personal Yoga mat, rug, or towel. Treat your meditation objects with respect, and you will make them sacred.

IT'S TOO NOISY

Noise can be a distraction from any Yoga practice. Sometimes, in the afternoons, instead of meditating on my inner peace, I sometimes find myself meditating on the neighbor's barking dog or leaf blower. As a result, I've found that the best time for me to meditate is before six in the morning, while most of the world is still sleeping peacefully. Swami Sivananda, the great sage of Rishikesh and my teacher's guru, actually said that we should be "up and doing" at four in the morning, because the vibrations at that hour are more conducive to meditation.

If you simply can't get up that early, though, and the noises of the day have already begun, try playing some peaceful meditative music. Ideally, this music will help block out the noise from the street but will not be too distracting. Swamiji, my beloved teacher, once suggested that I create a meditation CD. I named it "Omniscient Om" and recorded myself repeating "om" over a piano improvisation. Now, every time I put it on, the recording envelops me in a bubble of peaceful vibrations. I also like to listen to ambient music that is soothing and unobtrusive. I am a big fan of Telefon Tel Aviv and Bonobo.

MY KIDS COME IN WHEN I'M TRYING TO DO YOGA

That's great! You can begin to teach them Yoga, too! It's really important to give children an opportunity to experience a peaceful state. Their worlds are full of commotion, hurry, and noise, and by giving them a simple Yoga practice of their own, you will be doing them a big favor by giving them lifelong tools for relaxation and self-care.

Another option you have is to let your children make up their own prayers. It's okay to play with the divine! Those of us who grew up in the Judeo-Christian tradition are accustomed to thinking that there is only one God, but in the Eastern religions, there are many names and forms of God. For instance, one of the things I love about the Hindu tradition is the way they see God in everything! Your kids will love the colorful stories about the different Hindu gods. There's Lord Ganesha, who has the body of a man and the head of an elephant; Hanuman, the monkey god, who is known for his great strength; and Lord Nataraj, who is half-man, half-woman, and dances in a ring of fire!

Other mothers have told me that they keep a special basket full of toys and quiet activities to be used only during mommy's Yoga time. Figure out what works for your family, and begin enjoying Yoga with your children.

I'M TOO STIFF

If you eat at fast food restuarants, go everywhere by car, smoke cigarettes, or drink alcohol frequently, you may not be feeling so great. Lack of exercise, a toxic diet, and a fast-paced lifestyle can put stress on your body, leaving you stiff and achy. But don't let this put you off your Yoga practice! The physical poses will help to squeeze toxins out of the body and loosen things up. In addition, the breathing practices will help to purify the blood, removing toxins at a more subtle level.

You have to start somewhere. If you're stiff, so be it. In Yoga, you learn to accept your body as it is and love it anyway. Moreover, the body has amazing healing capabilities, and regular Yoga practice can stimulate and accelerate them. As I explained earlier, Yoga can be a powerful tool for increasing your health and wellness. If you can get yourself to practice it regularly, all that stiffness may just melt away! Given the proper opportunities, the body has a natural ability to correct itself. And with just a little effort, the body will start to come around. The ancient Vedic scriptures say, *Mana eva manushyanam karanam bandhamokshayoh*— "If you think you are bound, you are bound. If you think you are free, you are free." So have faith.

I CAN'T FIND YOGA CLOTHING IN MY SIZE

In the past, it was sometimes difficult to find Yoga clothes that fit in popular department stores. These days, more and more clothing and sporting good stores carry Yoga clothes in every size. What's more, we can all find clothes that fit through the internet. The internet makes it simple to find and purchase anything you might not otherwise be able to get locally. You can easily go online and find everything you need for your Yoga practice. Check out Old Navy, Target, Catherine's, and Junonia—you'll have lots of options.

I HAVE HEALTH ISSUES

Many people who are new to Yoga have some health issues. Maybe your health issues are the reason why you picked up this book in the first place. In a way, though, pain and ill health can be your friends, if they are responsible for convincing you to take action and and provide better care for yourself. You can either let your maladies rule your life, or you can take control of them. Yoga is a gentle and effective way to begin improving your physical and mental well-being. So congratulations to you for taking the first step!

Although you should always consult with a healthcare professional before undertaking a new exercise program, most health problems will not prevent you from doing an easy Yoga practice. Whether you're stiff from arthritis or on medication for high blood pressure or diabetes, you can still find your way to the mat or chair for a regular Yoga session. And over time, you will begin to notice your conditions improving.

The poses in *Big Yoga for Less Stress* will help tone the glands, organs, and endocrine system, and promote greater peace and stress relief. Regardless of your health status, make sure to check in with yourself regularly. No one knows your body as well as you do, and good body awareness can go a long way toward helping you avoid injury.

I CAN'T AFFORD TO GO TO A REGULAR CLASS

These days, the costs of attending Yoga classes can quickly add up, especially if you're a beginner and really want to immerse yourself in learning. The good news is, you don't need to take classes to learn the stress-reducing exercises in this book! The poses, breath work, and meditations described here can be done wherever and whenever you like—at home, in the office, in the airport.

If you decide to advance your practice, however, there are a number of ways to avoid racking up charges. Sometimes, Yoga studios will give you a good deal if you buy a month's worth of classes, so be sure to ask around. Signing up for a program is also a good incentive to keep up your practice. Alternatively, if you aren't employed full time, you might offer *seva*, or service, to the the studio in exchange for classes.

> "Tension is who you think you should be. Relaxation is who you are."
> —CHINESE PROVERB

Although there really isn't any substitute for an inspiring teacher, sometimes it just isn't possible or practical to find one close to you. If that is the case, go out and buy a new or used Yoga DVD, or borrow one from your local library. Then, watch and study it a few times before practicing. This may sound silly, but you will get some benefits simply through observation! Once you feel you have the hang of the poses, try doing the class along with the video. After a while you won't even need to look at the TV. You will will be able to just listen, draw your awareness in, and have a beautiful, meditative experience.

I'M OVERWHELMED BY MY EMOTIONS

At certain points in our lives, we get caught in emotional webs of anger and resentment and can't seem to find our way out. Or we find ourselves with hurt feelings because someone treated us unkindly. When we harbor negative emotions, it can be hard to settle down and practice Yoga. So what can we do? Thankfully, the Yogis have thought of everything. In the Yoga Sutras, Patanjali discusses how to calm the mind when it's churning with emotion. Book 1, Sutra 33, states:

"By cultivating attitudes of friendliness to the happy, compassion toward the unhappy, delight in the virtuous, and disregard for the wicked, the mindstuff retains its undisturbed calmness."

Swami Satchidananda elaborated on Patanjali's basic message, and called these attitudes the four locks and the four keys. Any time you come across a "lock," apply the proper "key" and you can keep your mind calm. In other words, when you meet a happy person, what's the best way to act? Jealous? No. Simply be friendly and enjoy that person's happiness. There's no need to try to bring a happy person down if you're feeling low yourself. And what about meeting an unhappy person? Does Patanjali suggest you try to offer him or her advice or cheer? No. Have compassion. If that unhappy person asks you for something and you can give it, that's okay, too. But you shouldn't feel that you have to "fix" him or her. If you're fortunate enough to meet a truly virtuous person, delight in his or her presence and maybe try to cultivate the virtuous qualities that you admire most. Remember, the whole point of the four locks and the four keys is to keep your mind calm.

And finally, what about the person who makes your blood boil? This is the real challenge. Do your best to disregard that person. Although it's not as easy as it sounds, it's a profound practice for strengthening the mind. You don't have to like everybody when you're a Yogi, but you can have compassion even for those who treat you badly. That being said, there's nothing wrong with staying away from people you don't like.

I have found these locks and keys to be a great comfort during stressful times, although they can apply to almost every situation. Often by simply meditating on my problems with compassion and equanimity, I find that solutions present themselves effortlessly. So instead of avoiding Yoga when you're upset, embrace it! Yoga will help you sort out your emotions and clear your mind.

I DON'T THINK I CAN DO THIS

I have never had a student who didn't have some body issues, no matter how thin, young, or beautiful she was. So don't be surprised if or when your mind starts telling you all the reasons why you can't do Yoga. It may be that you have reservations about your ability to do some of the poses found in this book. But don't let that stop you! You don't need to be a Yoga master to benefit from the moves I show you. As I've explained, the techniques and exercises in Part Two are easy, and can give extraordinary stress relief to anyone, from the newest beginner to the most experienced Yogi.

No matter what your ability level is, bring yourself to this ancient practice and listen to your body. Stretch to the edge of your comfort zone and rest there, paying conscious attention to the breath. The breath work I show you will give you a beautiful moment of stillness, and I won't have to tell you what a delicious feeling that is. Like the sensation of eating a juicy, ripe peach, the benefits of Yoga cannot be described. You have to experience them for yourself.

Besides any physical reservations you might have, you might feel you have some bad habits that are keeping you from doing Yoga. You might think that before you begin your Yoga practice, you need to give up smoking, drinking, overeating, purging, or other behaviors you might you label as "bad." While we should all strive to eliminate unhealthy habits, don't put off doing Yoga because you feel you're not ready. As part of your Yoga practice, begin to neutralize the judgments you make about your behaviors. You are exactly as God intended you to be. Go ahead and introduce Yoga into your life, and gradually you will develop such a love for your new, "good" habit that you won't feel so eager to indulge in your old ways.

STAY STRONG!

It can be difficult to make and maintain a lifestyle change such as a new fitness routine or diet. Sometimes it seems like you're taking one step forward and two steps back. Despite the obstacles you may encounter, have patience with yourself and don't give up. You'll receive so many benefits from doing Yoga just a few times a week that it's worthwhile to press through your lethargic tendencies. And as I mentioned earlier, you don't have to do every pose every day!

It's a good idea to alternate your routines so you don't get bored. In addition, you may want to vary the settings in which you practice Yoga. Take some time and determine which setting works best for you. For instance, instead of doing your Yoga practice on your own, you might prefer to team up with a friend or neighbor so you can encourage each other.

Personally, I find that when I need a Yoga tune-up, I receive the most inspiration from spending time at a Yoga ashram. It's like Yoga camp! Many contemporary ashrams offer month-long teacher training programs and private retreats for various lengths of time. Ashrams usually provide regularly scheduled meditations, classes, delicious vegetarian meals, and chanting sessions. Also, they offer the opportunity to socialize with other Yoga students and teachers and build supportive relationships. You can find a list of Yoga ashrams in the Resources section at the back of the book.

The important thing is that you do whatever it takes to keep up with your Yoga. Stick to your goals, and don't get frustrated and end up throwing in the towel. Set aside the time to make Yoga part of your lifestyle. After a while, the day may even come where you really miss your Yoga if you don't do it! Ultimately, Yoga is about disciplining your mind and body to achieve the greater goal of feeling peaceful, calm, and useful—not just on the mat, but all throughout your life.

LET'S GET STARTED!

Hopefully, reading Part One has encouraged you to commit to carving out some time to take better care of yourself. In Part Two, I will introduce you to a variety of Yoga practices that will allow you to reduce and even eliminate the stress from your life. Remember—you don't have to be thin to enjoy the benefits of Yoga. To underline this point, each of the poses and exercises in Part Two is demonstrated by a big, proud woman: me! By allowing Yoga into your life, you, too, can enjoy greater health and peace of mind than ever before.

Yoga Practices

Now that you've learned a little about the history and practice of Yoga, you're probably ready to try it out for yourself. In Part Two, I will introduce you to a number of basic techniques that can be used to help you relax and reduce your stress levels. The Yoga postures and sequences, breathing practices, and meditation described here are easy to learn and even easier to work into your busy day.

Chapter 5 provides you with some simple Yoga sequences that combine dynamic movements and more static postures. These sequences can be done almost anywhere—at home, at work, or at school. I begin with a chair-based routine, for those of you who want to be able to practice Yoga at your desks. You'll also learn a standing sequence to help you build strength. Finally, there is a special "Flex-Ability" sequence, which will tone the muscles that support your joints and simultaneously release toxins from your system. These straightforward stretches are ideal for anyone who is getting back into shape.

Chapter 6 will show you the ins and outs of the breathing practices known as *pranayama*. Pranayama provides a bridge between the body and the mind. The idea is that if you can control your breath, you can control your mind. The subtle yet powerful practices of pranayama bring fresh oxygen and *prana,* the life force, into every cell, eliminating toxins and re-energizing all the systems in your body. Conscious breathing also increases awareness of your thoughts and actions, helping you lead a life of emotional clarity and calm. I've given you a number of different simple breathing techniques that will help you to either relax or revitalize your entire body.

And in Chapter 7, I will teach you how to meditate. Meditation is a wonderful way to bring your mind and body into peace. In addition to showing you a basic meditation technique, I have provided a number of different meditations, each geared toward relieving a specific source of stress—grief, problems with loved ones, illness or injury, and money issues. That way, you can tailor your meditation practice to fit your daily needs.

Throughout Part Two, I've included pictures to help guide you. My goal with these images is not only to show you how to do these exercises, but also to prove that anybody can do them, regardless of size or shape! You don't have to be a supermodel to get into Yoga—Yoga rewards each of us equally.

When done regularly, Yoga poses, breathing practices, and meditation can be enormously effective in helping to control and even eliminate stress. You may even feel the benefits after a single session of physical postures. With so much to gain from these valuable techniques, why not get started right now?

Chapter Five

Yoga Poses for Stress Relief

In this chapter, I will show you three different sequences of Yoga poses to help you unwind and minimize the stiffness that develops when you are chronically stressed out. Developed from basic Hatha Yoga asanas, these poses are so simple that even a beginner will be able to perform them! What's more, you can do these exercises anywhere and at any time, so that it's no trouble to schedule a round into your day.

The first routine is done seated, so that you can perform it at home or even at your office desk. Your body will be so happy to have a forward bend or a side twist to wake up your spine in the middle of your work day! Think of your spine as a command center—it protects your spinal cord, which connects your brain to the rest of your body. The bends and twists in this sequence help move fresh blood into muscles that support the spine, invigorating the spinal cord and helping to reduce stress at the physical level. Other poses in the sequence open the upper chest area and bring new oxygen into the lungs, counteracting any tightness that may have developed in hunching over the computer. Overall, this simple sequence will re-energize all the systems in your body, bringing you back into balance.

The second routine is an adaptation of a more traditional standing sequence, *surya namaskar*, which translates into "the salute to the sun." It's ideal for building strength in the legs, expanding the lungs to bring in more revitalizing oxygen, and moving the spine in different directions—forward and back, and side to side.

Often, when we're feeling stressed, we collapse into ourselves, shoulders slumping and back slouching. This sequence will open up the chest and get you breathing again, turning off the stress response. I recommend that you do the salute to the sun at home or at the office.

Finally, the third routine is something I call the "Flex-Ability" series. As the name implies, this sequence combines movement with controlled breathing to help you improve your range of motion, working through each joint in your body. Flexibility is a key to living a life of ease, and the dynamic movements in this sequence will help you erase any stiffness that may be keeping you from other physical activity. The Flex-Ability series also helps you cultivate your awareness, getting you to pay attention to your internal bodily sensations as they arise and change from moment to moment. Neuroscientists call this consciousness of your inner sensations "interoception." I encourage you to do this sequence at home, so that you can really tune in to your body, getting more intimate with it in every session. In addition, a flexible body is better prepared to sit comfortably for meditation, which you'll learn about in Chapter 7. Actually, the ancient Yogis developed the physical practices of Yoga primarily as a way to increase their capacity to meditate for longer periods of time without discomfort.

The number of times you'll repeat each exercise in the sequence will vary. Some of the exercises only require one or two repetitions, while others should be repeated several times before moving on to the next. I've indicated the number of repetitions for each exercise and sequence in this chapter.

I recommend practicing each sequence all the way through to familiarize yourself with the flow of the poses and movements involved. Once you know each routine, though, you don't have to do the entire sequence in a single session. Sometimes it's easier to do a few of the exercises, work a little, then do a few more. As the stretches become more automatic, you can mix them up according to your needs. If you're hunching over a computer at work, for example, one of the back bend poses can help to break up the tension in the shoulders and neck. You may find that some of the movements become favorites, and that's fine. It's your body's way of telling you what you need.

Each sequence can be done by itself. You don't need to do all three sequences in a row—in fact, I advise against this. Instead, if you have time, finish your stretching routine with pranayama and/or meditation. This will bring about an even more profound sense of relaxation.

Please be kind to yourself as you approach these routines. It's best not to overdo it. Never force yourself into a position that is uncomfortable or painful. Whenever you feel discomfort, dial down the intensity and approach the pose more gently. Remember, you'll get the best results when you stay relaxed in your practice. Avoid building up tension. Whenever you feel your muscles start to tighten too much, have a little wiggle to invite them to relax. That said, don't bounce into a stretch. Instead, think of the body melting as you deepen the pose.

If you are recovering from an injury or simply haven't made time for exercise in the past, you may feel that you can't do the poses as they're shown in the pictures. Remember, it's not necessary to do a pose perfectly in order to benefit from it. As long as you stay relaxed and focus on your breathing, you will quickly start to feel better. Over time, you'll be able to improve your technique. In Yoga, we look for the sweet spot between effort and ease, so go to the edge if you like, but then back off a bit. Keep exploring, and enjoy the journey!

Seated Sequence

This first sequence is ideal for the office, or for anywhere you have to work in one position for a long period of time. This sequence counteracts the risk of repetitive stress injuries that comes with having a desk job. After a few hours spent staring at your computer, your body may feel tense and tight. By stretching and relaxing, and by breathing deeply with each movement, you increase blood flow to your muscles, organs, glands and heart. This helps re-energize your tired and cramped body. Moreover, by shifting your attention away from your work—an area over which you may not have much control—and bringing your focus inward to your body, you can help center, calm, and empower yourself.

 1. Crab Claw

 6. Warrior

 2. OMG

 7. Chair Twist

 3. Shoulder Blade Squeeze

 8. Chair Forward Bend

 4. Rock the Baby

 9. Chair Backward Bend

 5. Butterfly

STARTING POSITION

One of the nice things about this sequence is that it can be done without ever leaving your chair. Each exercise begins from a simple sitting pose. Sit forward on your chair, positioning yourself close to the front or side edge. Your feet should rest flat on the floor, about hips' width apart. If your legs are short or don't naturally reach the floor, you might want to put a bolster or pillow under your feet to make this pose more comfortable.

Throughout the sequence, be aware of your posture. Often, we tend to hunch over our desks, putting stress on our joints and ligaments and bringing our bones out of alignment. Keep your spine long and your shoulders wide, opening up your upper body. Imagine that your head is resting on top of your spine, and that the back of your neck is soft. Your neck should be as free and wiggly as a bobblehead doll's!

Tip: In Yoga, we try to balance the two sides of the body. So, any time you work one side of the body, you'll want to work the other side, too.

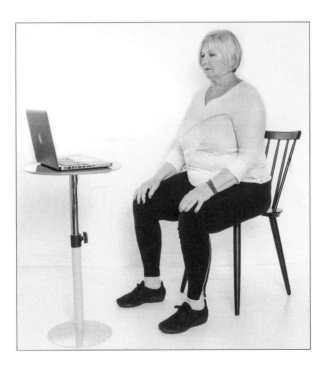

1. Crab Claw

BENEFITS

This exercise increases circulation in your fingers and alleviates joint pain there.

TECHNIQUE

Inhale as you splay your fingers wide. Exhale, curling your fingers into the shape of a claw, tensing all the muscles in your hand as tightly as is comfortable.

REPETITIONS

Four to eight. Notice that with each repetition, your joints will be able to bend a little bit more. Finish by wiggling all your fingers.

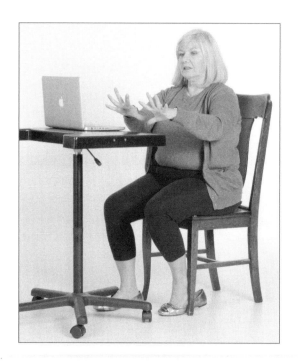 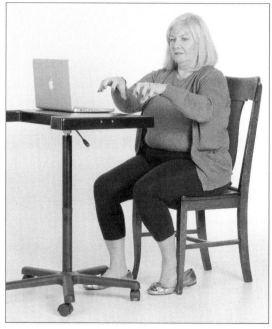

2. OMG

BENEFITS

This exercise increases circulation to your facial muscles, preventing or alleviating headaches. It also helps prevent wrinkles!

TECHNIQUE

Inhale as you raise your eyebrows, open your eyes wide, open your mouth, and stick out your tongue. Hold your breath for as long as is comfortable, then exhale, scrunching up your face like a prune.

REPETITIONS

One to three. Finish by closing your eyes and relaxing your face completely.

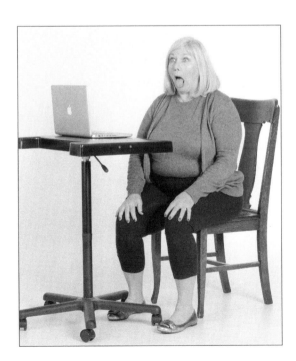 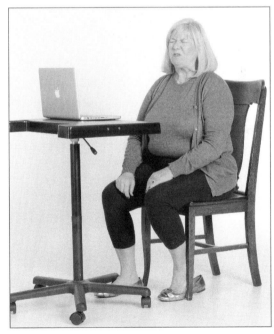

3. Shoulder Blade Squeeze

BENEFITS

This exercise offsets the constant hunching of the shoulders that plagues desk workers, preventing stiffness and back- and neck-ache.

TECHNIQUE

Inhale as you bring your hands behind your head, interlacing your fingers. Relax your shoulders so they don't inch up toward your ears. Exhale as you squeeze your shoulder blades together behind you, imagining your elbows pointing toward each other, as if they could touch behind your back. This is one repetition. Keep the hands interlaced as you inhale for the next round, releasing the shoulder blade squeeze. Exhale as you continue, bringing your elbows backward and squeezing the area between your shoulder blades.

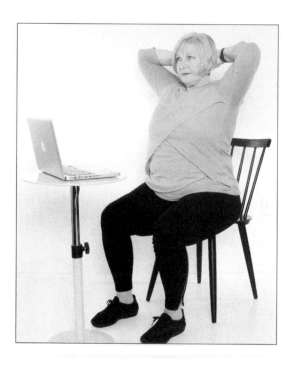 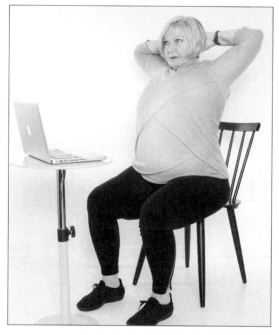

REPETITIONS

Three to five.

Intermediate: To go deeper in this stretch, bend to your right side as you exhale and squeeze your shoulder blades together. Return to the starting position as you inhale, and then bend to your left side on your next exhale. This is one round.

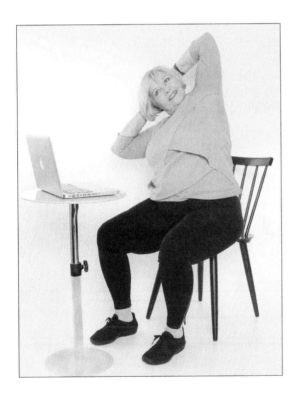
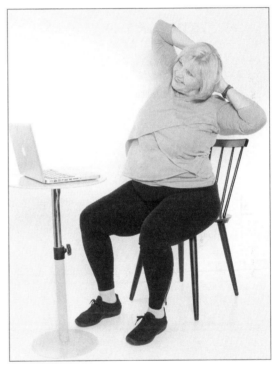

4. Rock the Baby

BENEFITS

This exercise stretches and tones the muscles that support your hips, and brings more blood to the hip joints.

TECHNIQUE

Inhale and raise your right knee, using your hands if necessary. Exhale and cradle your right foot in your left hand. Your right hand will cradle your right knee in the same manner. Continue to breathe normally as you gently lift your right leg up a few inches and rock it from side to side. Repeat on the other side. This constitutes one repetition.

REPETITIONS

One or two, rocking each leg gently for as long as you're comfortable.

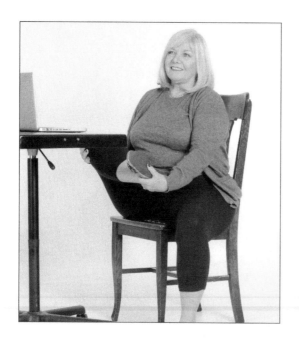 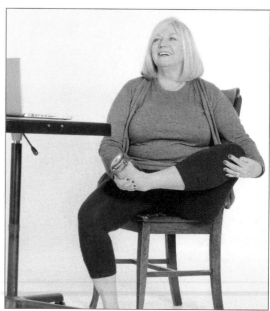

5. Butterfly

BENEFITS

This exercise alleviates sciatica, improves circulation to the hip joint, and is good for digestion.

TECHNIQUE

As in the previous exercise, inhale and raise your right knee. Exhale, placing your right ankle on your left knee and supporting your right foot with your left hand. Continue breathing normally as you lay your right hand softly on your right knee and gently bounce the knee up and down for as long as is comfortable. Bring the foot back to the floor on an exhalation. Repeat on the other side to complete one round. To finish, return to the simple sitting pose and relax, noticing the effects of the stretch.

REPETITIONS

One or two.

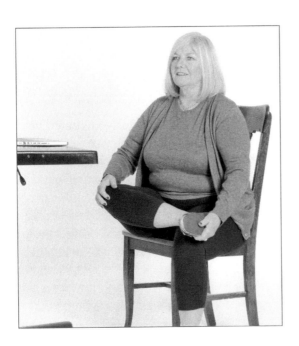
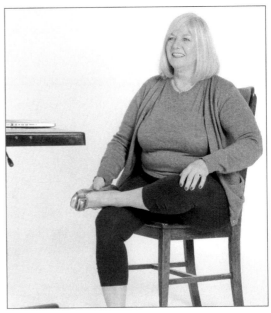

6. Warrior

Virabhadrasana

BENEFITS

This exercise builds leg strength, opens your chest for deeper breathing, and improves the alignment of your hips and shoulders.

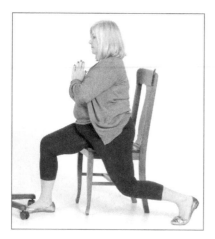

TECHNIQUE

Shift your position so that you are seated toward the left side of the chair. Stretch your left leg behind you, shin parallel to the floor. Your left foot will be flexed, forming a right angle with the floor, toes rooted to the mat and heel lifted. Bring your hands together at the heart center—that is, at chest level, as if in prayer. This hand position is called *anjali mudra*. (See inset on next page.) Take a deep breath in and out. Then, bring your hands back to your lap and return to the simple sitting pose. Repeat the sequence on your other side: shift to the right side of the chair and stretch your right leg behind you, bringing your hands into anjali mudra.

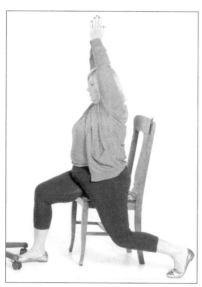

REPETITIONS

Hold each position for a few breaths, and do up to three repetitions.

Advanced: To deepen the stretch, after you stretch your left leg back, inhale and move your hands over your head, keeping them folded in anjali mudra. Take care to keep your shoulders from hunching up. Feel the activation of energy in your arms, the sense of lightness in the pose. Hold the position for a few breaths, then exhale as you bring your hands back to your chest. Focus on your heart center for a moment, then release your hands, letting them come back to your lap. Come back to the simple sitting pose and repeat the sequence, extending the other leg behind you. To finish, return to the simple sitting pose.

Mudras

The Sanskrit word *mudra* means "sign" or "seal," and can be understood as a sacred or symbolic gesture seen in Hindu and Buddhist religious practices. In the Yogic tradition, mudras are said to produce a kind of electrical current within the body, helping to bring about an inner state of aliveness. There are many different mudras. Although mudras can engage different parts of the body, most are completed with the hands. The mudra practiced in the warrior pose and in the salute to the sun is called anjali mudra. In anjali mudra, you bring your hands together at chest level, aligning them with your heart center. This mudra is considered a form of salutation and is often accompanied by the word "namaste." If someone greets you with anjali mudra and "namaste," she is saying, "I bow to the divinity in you from the divinity within me."

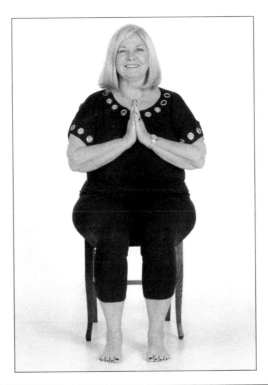

7. Chair Twist

BENEFITS

Twists help refresh the spine, increasing blood circulation there; they also benefit the pancreas, kidneys, and adrenal glands.

TECHNIQUE

From the starting position, inhale and feel your spine lifting. Exhale and twist to the left, bringing your left arm behind you to take hold of the back of the chair. Your right hand will cross over to rest on your left knee. Turn your head to the left, keeping the bottom of your chin parallel to the floor. To come out of the stretch, lead with your head, and return to the starting position carefully and deliberately. Repeat on the other side to complete one round.

REPETITIONS

Up to three rounds. Hold the twist for three to five breaths, twisting a little further on the exhalations, and feeling the spine lifting on the inhalations.

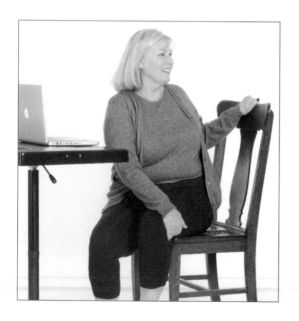 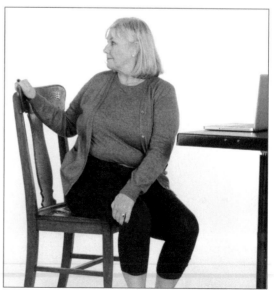

8. Chair Forward Bend

BENEFITS

This exercise lengthens and aligns your spine, gives a massage to the internal organs, and increases your awareness of your breathing.

TECHNIQUE

In the starting position, exhale and bend forward at your hips. You can glide your hands down your legs for support, or you can simply reach forward and down toward your feet or the pillow, going only as far as you can without straining. Let your head relax and the back of your neck soften. Rest here and breathe naturally for up to five breaths. Enjoy the sensation of the gentle rising and falling of the torso with each inhale and exhale. Then inhale once more and come back to the starting position, bringing your palms to rest on your lap. Close your eyes and feel the effects of the forward bend.

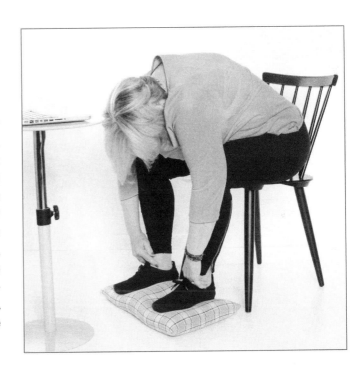

REPETITIONS

Three to five.

Tip: If this move is uncomfortable because you carry a little extra abdominal weight, widen your stance to make a well for the belly as you lower yourself down. Alternatively, shorten the length of time you hold the pose. It's more important that you stay relaxed than that you hold the position for a long time. Remember, you can always do another round.

9. Chair Backward Bend

BENEFITS

This exercise squeezes the muscles that support the spine, increasing circulation in that area. It also opens the chest, expanding the heart and allowing the lungs to fill with fresh oxygen and prana.

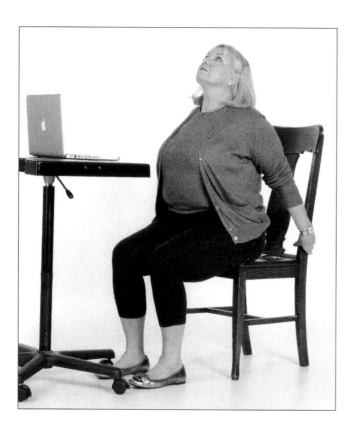

TECHNIQUE

Inhale and reach your hands behind you to hold the sides or back of the chair. Arch your spine, allowing your chest and breastbone to lift. Exhale, and relax a little. On the next inhalation, squeeze your shoulder blades together. Release the squeeze on the exhale. This is one round.

REPETITIONS

Three to six. Finish by gently dropping your chin to your chest to counteract and balance the stretch, then come back to simple sitting pose, hands on your lap.

How to Perform a Body Scan

At the end of your stretching sequence, I recommend that you do a relaxing scan of your whole body to release any tension left over from your practice. This sequence can be done while you're still seated in your chair. Here's how you do it:

Begin by giving your entire body a big squeeze. Tense every muscle in your body as tightly as you can. Lift your legs, raise your arms up a bit, and make fists. Hold this tension for a moment, and then release it. Imagine you're a rubber band that has been stretched out and suddenly let go. Do it one more time: tight, tight, tight—then release!

Now, with your feet resting twelve or more inches apart on the floor, place your hands comfortably on your lap and take a deep breath. Exhale and continue to breathe normally. With your eyes closed and your awareness drawn inward, become conscious of the soles of your feet. Notice any residual tension and let it melt away. Mentally, move to the tops of your feet, toes,

and arches, releasing any tension you may find in those areas.

Continue by observing your ankles, shins, calves, knees and thighs. Relax. Move your awareness to your palms, wrists, forearms, elbows and upper arms. Relax. Observe your belly as it rises and falls with each breath. Relax your hips, buttocks, and groin area. Relax your upper chest and your internal organs. Feel your back muscles letting go. Relax your shoulder blades and shoulders, neck, and all the parts of your head—from your chin, jaw, cheeks, lips, nose, eyes, eyebrows, forehead, all the way up to the crown of your head.

Pause for a few minutes as you enjoy the lightness of total relaxation. Give yourself a mental pat on the back for taking some time to bring your whole self into balance.

If you would like more guidance in performing your body scan, go to www.BigYogaForLessStress.com to download a free recording of the practice. Alternatively, feel free to use this script to record your own version of the body scan.

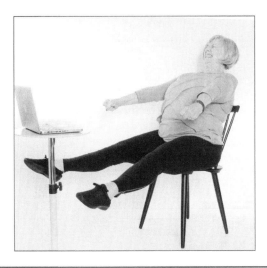

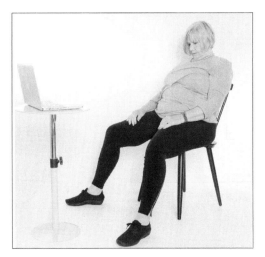

standing sequence

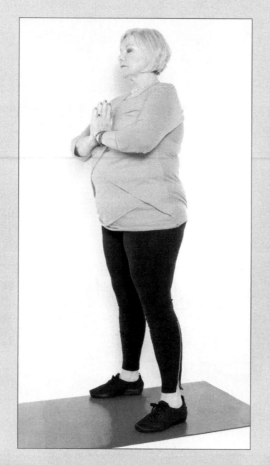

This next sequence is a wonderful way to get your blood moving during a long day at the office. It can be used as a pick-me-up when you're starting to feel tired or distracted. Done slowly and more deliberately, this sequence can also help calm you down after a stressful encounter with a colleague. Note that you will initiate each movement with an inhale or an exhale, but that you will continue to breathe as you explore and deepen each pose. For those who would like to see the sequence in motion, a version of this sequence can be found on the Big Yoga Flex-Ability DVD.

10. Salute to the Sun with Chair

Surya Namaskar, adapted

BENEFITS

The salute to the sun offers many physiological benefits. The lunges and the chair pose (*utkatasana*) help strengthen your leg muscles, and especially help protect the knee joints. In addition, the lunges open your pelvis and abdomen, providing more space for your internal organs to be refreshed with new blood. The forward bends bring blood to your brain and give a gentle massage to your internal organs. The back bends open the chest area, providing more space for your lungs to bring in more oxygen. And the gentle twists massage your digestive tract, helping to reduce stagnation.

REPETITIONS

Do each exercise in the sequence once before moving on to the next. Perform two or three rounds of the entire powerful sequence—or just one—according to your mood and capacity. Take all the time you need. Done quickly, the sun salutation can perk you up when you start to space out in the late afternoon. Or, if you're feeling jumpy and unsettled, this sequence can be done slowly to calm you down. Follow with a full body scan (see inset on page 59) and pranayama (see Chapter 6) if time permits.

CONSIDERATIONS

It's helpful to practice this sequence in bare feet and to use a sticky mat on the floor. Take care to ground your feet and use the chair to support you! These measures improve your traction, reducing the likelihood that you'll slip or lose your balance.

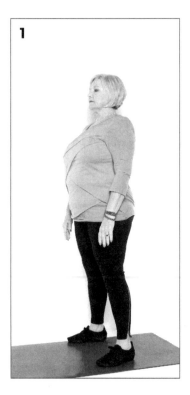
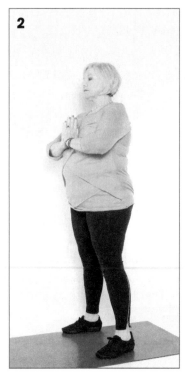
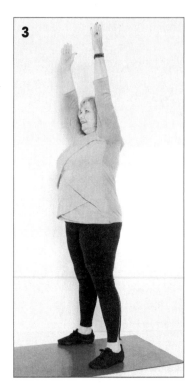

Position 1

Stand a little more than arms' length behind your chair. Your feet should be about a foot apart, directly under your hips. Your arms are at your sides, palms facing your thighs. You are now in *tadasana,* the mountain pose. Feel that you are steady and strong as a mountain. Relax deeply into your center, and tune in to the innate joy of your being.

Position 2

Inhale and bring your hands together in anjali mudra (see page 55) in front of your chest. Exhale, and feel yourself connecting with the earth.

Position 3

On the next inhale, drop your arms back to the sides of your body and then raise your arms up overhead. Your palms should be facing each other; alternatively, you can interlace your fingers.

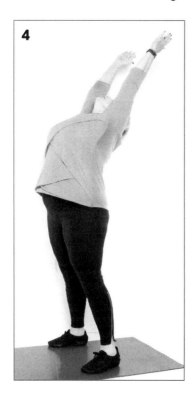
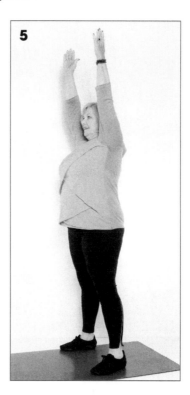

Position 4

Exhale and bend backwards, keeping your arms alongside your ears to protect your neck. Squeeze your shoulder blades together.

Position 5

Inhale and come out of your backbend, your arms over your head, palms facing each other.

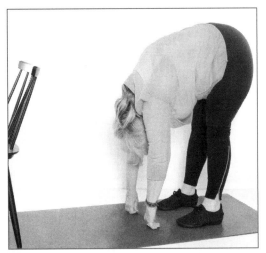

Position 6

Exhale and bend forward and down from the hips, allowing your arms to float downwards in a swan-dive motion. You can bend your knees to make this motion more comfortable. Soften your arms and the back of your neck in this standing forward bend. Take a few breaths here, and feel your spine lengthening.

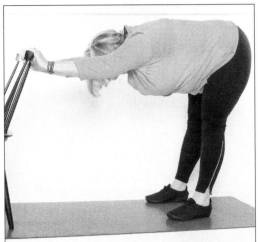

Position 7

Inhale and bring your hands to the top of the back of the chair. Your back should be parallel to the floor and your head should be between your arms, looking toward the floor. Imagine that a straight line extends from the top of your head to your tailbone. Knees can be straight or slightly bent—whichever is more comfortable for you. You are now in half-dog pose. Soften the back of your neck. Breathe deeply, and observe the movement of what we in Yoga refer to as the "side ribs"—the area of the rib cage directly under the armpit.

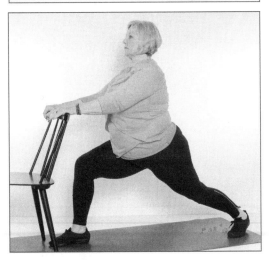

Position 8

Next is a lunge. Keeping your hands on top of the chair, inhale and step forward with your right foot, bringing it close to the chair. Sink into this lunge, breathing deeply. Be careful to keep your right knee directly above your right ankle—your leg should be bent at about a ninety-degree angle. Don't overextend your lunge, as you can hurt yourself if your knee pushes beyond your ankle here. Tuck your elbows into your torso to keep your shoulders from rising. As you lunge forward with your right foot, the heel of your back (left) foot will lift.

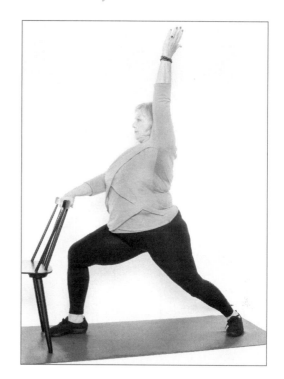

Position 9

Remaining in the lunge position, inhale and raise your left arm overhead, palm facing inward. Your right hand should stay on top of the chair, supporting you.

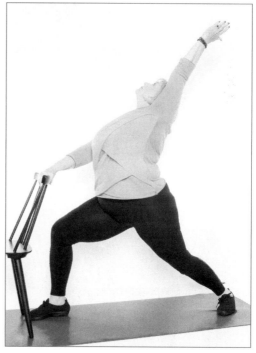

Position 10

Exhale and gently bend backward, keeping your left arm alongside your head. Breathe normally as you deepen your stretch.

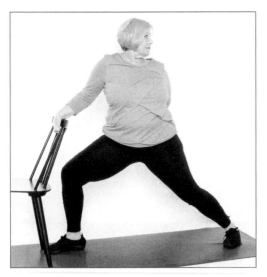

Position 11

On your next exhalation, come out of the back bend and return your left arm to your side. Twist to the left, bringing your left arm behind your back. Turn your head to look over your left shoulder, keeping your chin parallel to the floor. Breathe deeply, focusing on this spinal twist.

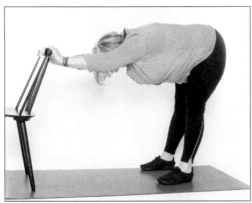

Position 12

Inhale and release the twist. Come back into the half-dog pose by bringing your right foot back to meet your left and bending forward at your hips. Place both hands on the top of the chair. Soften the back of your neck. Breathe deeply, and observe the movement of your side ribs as your lungs expand and contract with each inhalation and exhalation.

Now we're going to do the other side!

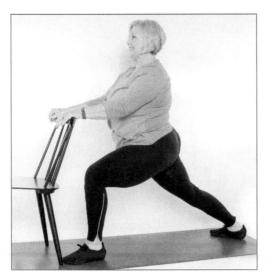

Position 13

Keeping your hands on top of the chair, inhale and lunge on your other side, stepping close to the chair with your left foot, left knee bent at a ninety-degree angle over your left ankle. Tuck your elbows into your torso to prevent your shoulders from rising. As you lunge forward with your left foot, the heel of your back (right) foot will lift up. Sink deeply into your lunge and take a breath or two.

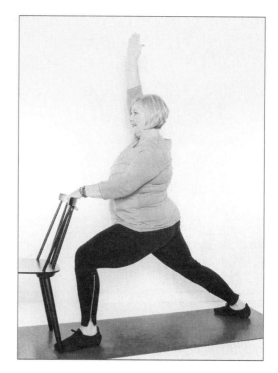

Position 14

Remaining in the lunge position, inhale and raise your right arm overhead, palm facing inward. Your left hand should stay on top of the chair, supporting you.

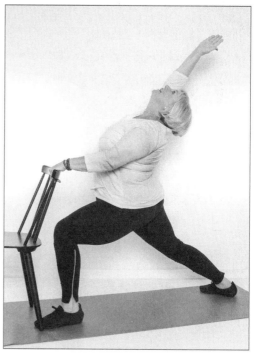

Position 15

Exhale and gently bend backward, keeping your right arm alongside your head. Concentrate on your breathing as you deepen your stretch.

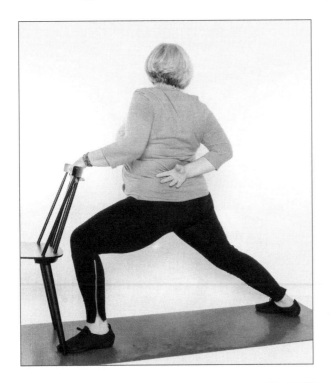

Position 16

On your next exhalation, come out of the back bend and return your right arm to your side. Twist to the right, bringing your right arm behind your back. Turn your head to look over your right shoulder, keeping your chin parallel to the floor. Remember to keep breathing!

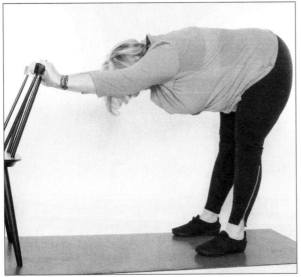

Position 17

On an exhale, release the twist slowly and deliberately. Bring your left foot back to meet your right. Bend forward at your hips and return both hands to the top of the chair. You are now back in half-dog pose again. Soften the back of your neck. Breathe deeply, and observe the movement of your side ribs as your lungs expand and contract with each inhalation and exhalation.

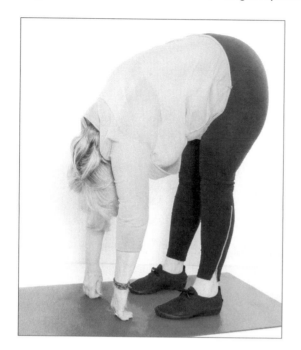
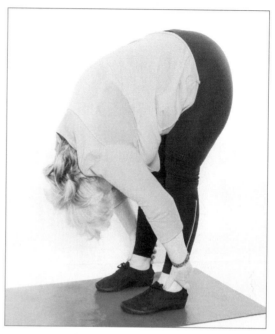

Position 18

Exhale and push away from the chair. Bend down and reach toward the floor with your fingertips, as if you were trying to touch your toes. But don't strain—imagine you are a rag doll. Soften your knees and allow your arms to hang freely. Alternatively, you may clasp your elbows and bring your head between your arms. This is a standing forward bend. To intensify the stretch, clasp your ankles and draw your head a little closer to your knees.

Position 19

Inhale and widen your stance so that your feet are about eighteen inches apart. Come into a squat: bend your knees and drop your buttocks. As you do, raise your arms to the level of your ears, palms facing each other. Don't let your knees cave in toward each other. Stay in the squat for as long as you like, breathing deeply.

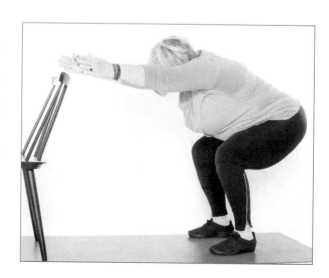

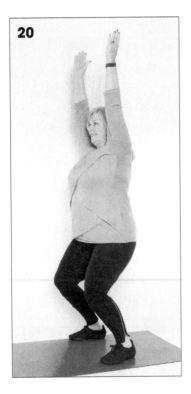 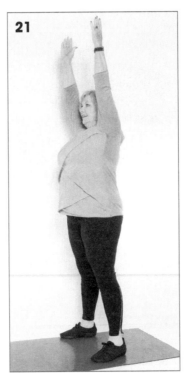 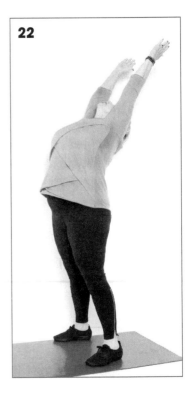

Position 20

Exhale and partially unbend your knees, coming about three-quarters of the way into a standing position. Keep your arms alongside your ears throughout. You are now in chair pose, or *utkatasana*—imagine that there is a chair behind you and you're about to sit down on it. Feel the strength of your thigh muscles as they contract, or activate, as we say in Yoga.

Position 21

Inhale and straighten your legs, bringing your arms overhead, palms facing each other. Drop your shoulders, please!

Position 22

Exhale and bend backward, focusing on your upper back. Keep your arms alongside your ears to protect your neck and squeeze your shoulder blades together.

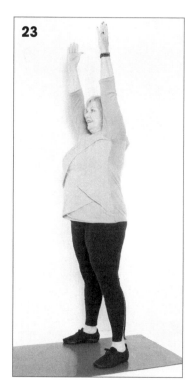
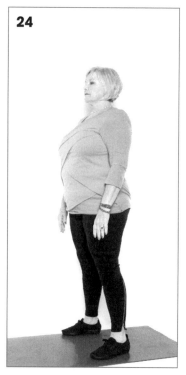
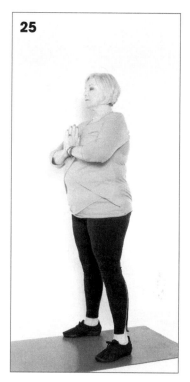

Position 23

Inhale and come back to a standing position, arms overhead. Your palms can face each other, or you can interlace your fingers.

Position 24

Exhale and float your arms out and downward, palms facing the earth, until they come to the sides of your body.

Position 25

Bring your palms back together in anjali mudra and close your eyes. Pause for a moment, breathing normally. Then drop your arms, adjust your feet to a comfortable stance, and relax as you observe the effects of the salute to the sun.

Flex-Ability Sequence

I learned this next sequence from my movement mentor, Hope Mell, who learned it from the founder of Structural Yoga Therapy, Mukunda Stiles, who adapted it from a sequence taught in the Bihar school of Yoga. I call this series a "Flex-Ability" sequence, because it improves your flexibility and thus also your ability to cope with stress. When your body is flexible, your mind will follow, enabling you to face your challenges and let unimportant worries roll off your back.

In the Flex-Ability sequence, stretches are done deliberately, at a snail's pace, as if you were moving in slow motion. Each of the movements is dynamic—that is, coordinated with your inhalations and exhalations—and not static, or fixed. As a result, the sequence simultaneously tones the muscles that support your joints and helps rid your joints of toxins. The breathing component of the sequence also brings more oxygen and prana into your body. Regular practice of the Flex-Ability series promotes a sense of lightness throughout your body.

This series is intended to be easy. It's a great introductory sequence for students who might find standard Hatha Yoga poses a bit challenging. The entire sequence is designed to be done on the floor, but can also be done seated in a chair, or even in bed. From start to finish, it can take as little as twenty-five minutes to complete. Don't feel you have to do the entire sequence all at once, though. It can be helpful to perform the sequence in chunks, doing ten minutes here, ten minutes there. To make the Flex-Ability sequence more effective for combating stress, follow it with a relaxing body scan (see page 59). Or, if you have more time, you can do a longer progressive relaxation (see pages 133 to 136), pranayama, or meditation. If you like, you can do it all—body scan, progressive relaxation, pranayama, and meditation—in that order.

Don't underestimate the power of the Flex-Ability series to effect positive change in your body!

11. Flex and Point

 12. Book Feet

 13. Ankle Circles

 14. Knee Bend

 15. Cat-Cow

 16. Hip Juicifier

 17. Extended Leg Pose

 18. The Dip

 19. Love Your Fingers

 20. Wrist Wrangling

 21. Figure Eights

 22. Elbow Bends

 23. Side Stretch

 24. Side Twist

 25. Upper Back Opener

 26. Scarecrow

 27. Forward & Backward Arch

 28. Shoulder Lubricator

 29. Say Yes!

 30. Say No!

 31. Curious Dog

STARTING POSITION

Most of these exercises start with you sitting on the floor in *dandasana,* or staff pose. Extend your legs in front of you, feet about twelve inches apart. Gently draw your shoulders up toward your ears, rotate them backward, and then release them. This will help open your chest and lift your sternum. Place your hands flat on the floor behind your body, or, if you prefer, you can rest your hands on your lap.

The entire sequence can also be done in a chair. I suggest learning the entire routine on the floor, if possible, and then using the same stretches throughout your day as you sit in your office chair. The breathing alone will bring more energy into your system, and the stretches will enliven your body.

As you perform the stretches, you should be conscious of your breath. Each inhalation should be performed deeply, through the nose. Your breaths should be full and noisy—that way, you won't forget to keep thinking about them! In contrast to most Yoga breathing, in the Flex-Ability series, you will be exhaling through your mouth. This allows you to get a more complete exhalation. You can enhance the benefits of the sequence by imagining that every inhalation is bringing in fresh prana and every exhalation is releasing toxins from your system.

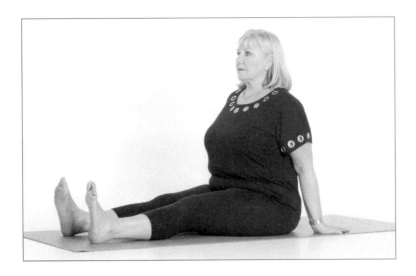

REPETITIONS

I recommend doing five to eight repetitions of each exercise before moving on to the next. Simply do as many repetitions as you can. Beginners, for example, will want to do fewer repetitions of each exercise. With practice, you can work up to more repetitions—eight repetitions is ideal.

11. Flex and Point

BENEFITS

Your feet form the foundation of your body—and it's important to keep your foundation strong! These stretches will help keep your ankles flexible. One of my students twisted her ankle recently, and she swears that she avoided serious injury because of her frequent practice of the Flex-Ability series.

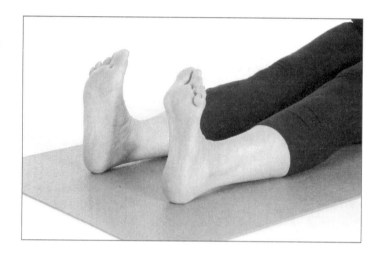

TECHNIQUE

Inhale and point your toes up toward the sky, splaying your toes and extending your heels away from the body. Exhale and point your toes forward. This is one repetition.

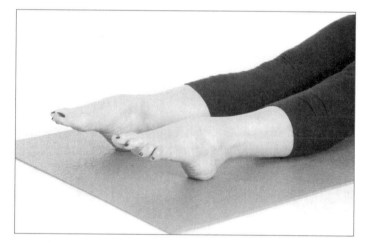

12. Book Feet

BENEFITS

We don't often think of our ankles as being capable of moving sideways, but they are! By building lateral strength in your ankles, you can help prevent injuries.

TECHNIQUE

With your heels on the floor, inhale and bring the balls of your feet together. Keeping your feet upright, exhale and bring the soles of your feet as close together as you can, as if you were closing a book. Inhale and open the feet again. This is one repetition.

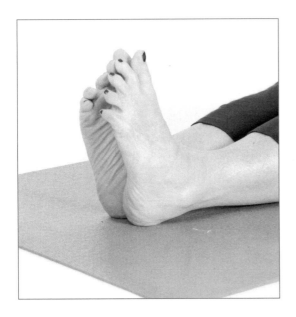 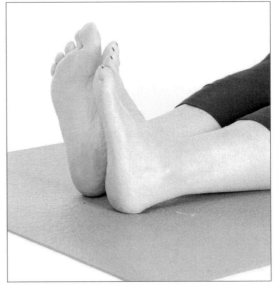

13. Ankle Circles

BENEFITS

This exercise increases ankle mobility and improves blood circulation to the feet.

TECHNIQUE

With your feet side by side, draw circles with your toes, bending from your ankles. Inhale as you go downward, and exhale coming upward. Do as many repetitions as you like in a clockwise direction, and do then do the same number of repetitions in a counterclockwise direction.

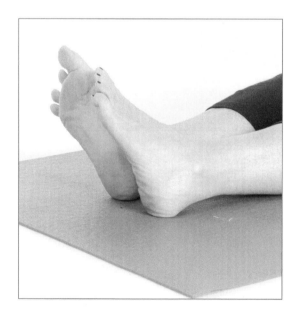 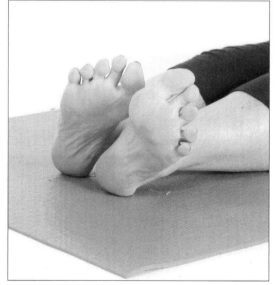

14. Knee Bend

BENEFITS

This stretch will give you a sense of the muscles that support the knees. When these muscles are weak, walking and other movements put stress on the corresponding joints in your knees, increasing your risk of injury.

TECHNIQUE

Beginning with an exhalation, draw your right knee up, clasping your hands under your right thigh for support. Then inhale and extend your right leg out in front of you and lift it about six inches off the ground, keeping your right foot soft. Imagine that your right foot, ankle, knee, and hip are connected by a straight line. On the exhalation, draw your right knee back up toward your chest. Repeat for as many times as is comfortable for you. Return to the starting position, bringing your right leg to rest on the floor next to your left leg. Now switch to your left leg, and perform the same number of repetitions as you did on the right leg.

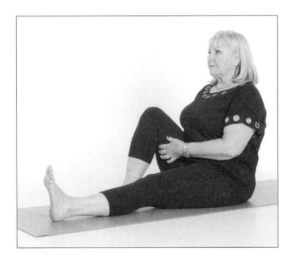
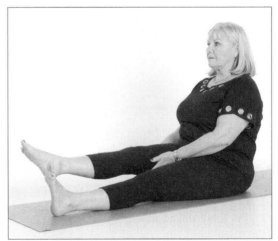

15. Cat-Cow

BENEFITS

This is an easy stretch that can be done throughout the day to wake up your spine and bring more oxygen and prana to your lungs.

TECHNIQUE

Start on your hands and knees. Your hands should be directly under your shoulders and your knees should be under your hips. Inhale. Exhale and arch your back, bringing your chin into your chest, tucking your tailbone under, and drawing your belly up toward your spine. This is the "cat" part of the pose. Next, inhale, drop your belly, and tilt your pelvis forward as if you were emptying a bowl. Lift your chin slightly, feeling a gentle squeeze at the back of your neck and across the bottom of your shoulder blades. This is the "cow" part of the pose. You have now completed one repetition.

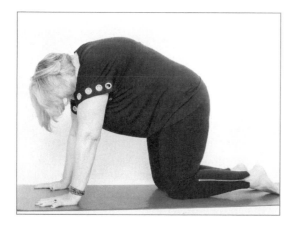 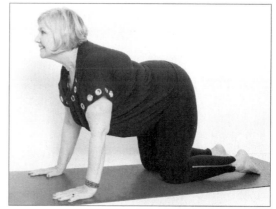

16. Hip Juicifier

BENEFITS

The hips help move us forward—literally! Is there some reason you're afraid to move ahead in your life? It may show up as pain in your hips. This exercise refreshes the synovial fluid within your hip joints, helping your bones glide effortlessly over each other. It also strengthens the muscles that support the hips.

TECHNIQUE

Spread your legs as wide apart as is comfortable. You may need to adjust your position so that your sit bones are grounded (see inset). Keep your balance by bracing yourself with your arms behind you, or, if you are performing this sequence in a chair, by holding the sides of the chair behind your buttocks. Inhale and turn the big toe of your right foot into the floor, raising your right hip slightly. Exhale and sweep your right leg over to meet your left, keeping the leg as straight as possible. Inhale and rotate your foot so that your right pinky toe touches the floor, and sweep the leg back to the wide stance. Complete as many repetitions as you like with your right leg, and then do the same number of repetitions with your left.

Grounding Your Sit Bones

The way you sit is critical to your Yoga practice. Whether you're performing certain poses, working on your breathing, or meditating, you'll find you need a firm, comfortable seat. And to attain this, you'll need to ground your sit bones. Your sit bones, or ischial tuberosities, are the lowest bones in your pelvis—they're the two curved bumps that you feel when you sit at the edge of a chair and tilt forward slightly. Ordinarily, if you're sitting correctly, you balance on these bones and use them to support your upper body. Your sit bones also help keep your spine properly aligned. Sometimes when you're moving around over the course of your Yoga practice, however, your ischial tuberosities lose contact with the surface on which you're sitting. You see, the flesh of your buttocks is great for cushioning your sit bones, but when it shifts around, it can prevent you from maintaining a steady, centered posture. To ground yourself and provide better access to your sit bones, you may want to gently move your buttock flesh out of the way before you perform certain poses.

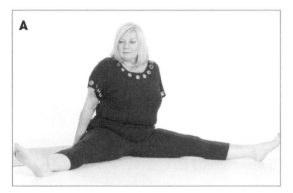

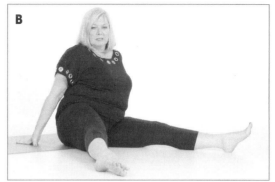

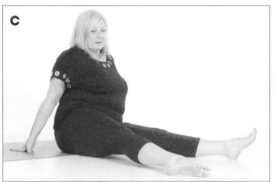

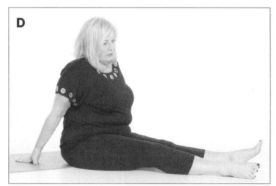

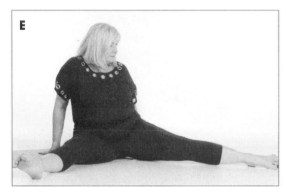

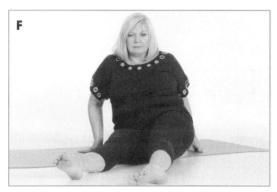

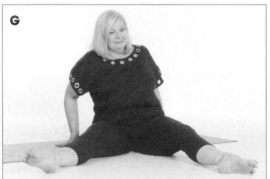

17. Extended Leg Pose

BENEFITS

This position builds strength in your legs. It also gives a gentle massage to your abdomen and elongates your spine.

TECHNIQUE

Begin on all fours, as you did in the cat-cow pose. Inhale and extend your right leg behind you. Lift your chin slightly, and keep your right foot soft—no need to point your toes. Your pelvic bones should be parallel to the floor and you should feel a slight lumbar curve, as in the cat-cow pose. As you exhale, draw your chin and knee toward each other under your chest, and arch your back like a cat. Do as many repetitions as you can on the right side before doing the same number of repetitions on the left side.

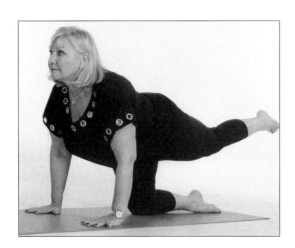 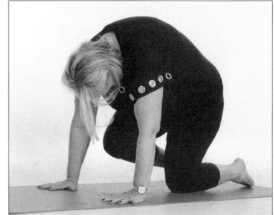

18. The Dip

BENEFITS

This exercise offers a great stretch for your sides, working muscles from your neck all the way down to your tailbone, and on both your right and your left sides.

TECHNIQUE

Begin on all fours, as in the cat-cow pose, but this time, bring your knees and legs together. Your hands should be placed a little more than shoulder width apart, and slightly in front of you—off your mat, if necessary. Inhale here, in neutral. Then exhale and dip your right hip, bringing it as close to the floor as is comfortable. Turn your head to the left to get a curve all along the entire length of your right side. Inhale and return to the neutral position. Then exhale as you rotate and dip to the left, turning your head toward the right for a great stretch. This is one repetition.

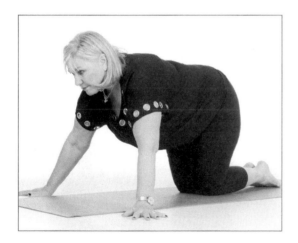 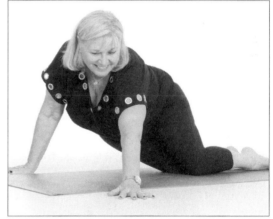

19. Love Your Fingers

BENEFITS

After being on your hands and knees for a few exercises, your wrists can feel a little uncomfortable. The stretch helps to counteract any wrist strain; it is also helpful when used to refresh the fingers after you have been typing too long.

TECHNIQUE

Sit in any comfortable position, such as dandasana or *vajrasana* (thunderbolt pose), as pictured here (see inset on next page). Stretch your arms out in front of you, fingers pointing toward the sky. Inhale and splay your fingers wide, keeping your shoulders from inching up. Exhale and curl your fingers downward, toward your wrists. This is one repetition.

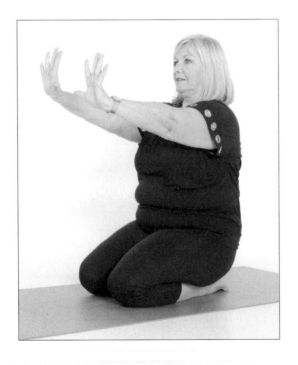
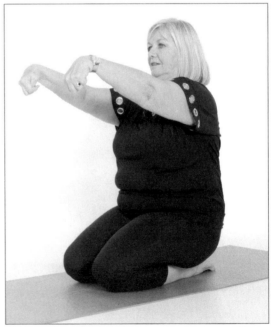

Vajrasana

Vajrasana, the thunderbolt pose, is excellent for the digestion. It also encourages flexibility in the hips, legs, and knees. To assume the vajrasana pose, sit with your heels tucked under you and your shins and the tops of your feet pressed against the floor. While it may not be comfortable for you at first, I highly recommend getting into the habit of using this pose. The pose is beneficial even if you can only maintain it for five seconds, and it will become easier over time.

If you want to make the pose more comfortable, adapt it by putting a cushion under the hips or ankles, or behind the knees. You can also use a small meditation bench to gently coax the thigh muscles to relax, as in the picture here.

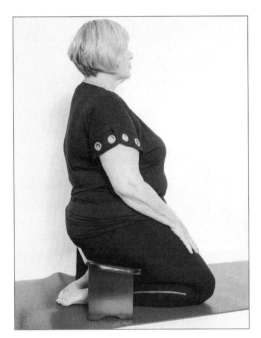

Sukhasana

Sukhasana, or easy pose, is an excellent resting pose for many of the exercises in this section. Simply cross your right leg in front of your left. If this is uncomfortable, slide a pillow or bolster under your knees to allow your hips to relax. Alternatively, a pillow can be placed under your buttocks to lift your hips a little higher than your knees. Once you get used to it, sukhasana is also a great pose for meditation because of the stability it offers you. It also creates an openness in the body, allowing energy to flow freely.

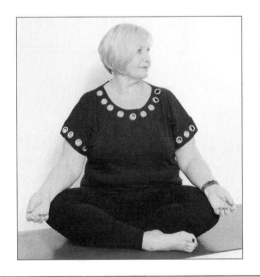

20. Wrist Wrangling

BENEFITS

This exercise also helps increase wrist mobility.

TECHNIQUE

Sit in any comfortable position—you can use dandasana, sukhasana (see inset on page 85), or vajrasana here. Keeping your elbows tucked into your sides, bring your hands out in front of you, palms up. Inhale and bring the sides of your pinkies together, as if you were reading a book. Keep your palms as flat as possible. Exhale and rotate your hands at the wrist, so that the tips of your middle fingers are touching. Maintain the flatness of your palms; your elbows should stay tucked in. This is one repetition.

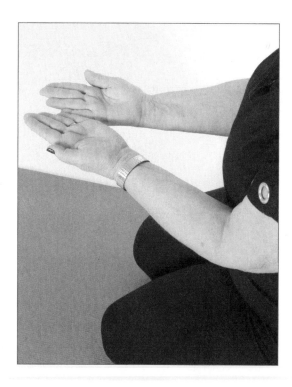 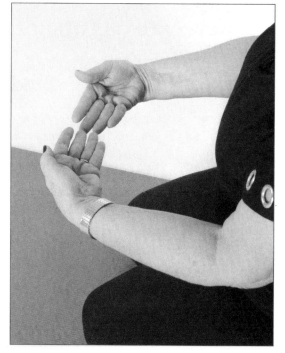

21. Figure Eights

BENEFITS

This exercise helps prevent carpal tunnel syndrome. It also increases blood circulation to your wrists.

TECHNIQUE

Sitting in any comfortable position, make two gentle fists in front of you. While holding your fists together, begin making slow figure eights, inhaling as your fists move downward and exhaling as your fists move upward. Do as many repetitions as you feel comfortable doing, then do the same number of repetitions tracing your figure eights in the opposite direction. It might be a little confusing to draw your eights backward, but you'll soon get the hang of it! Do as many figure eights in this direction as you did for the first.

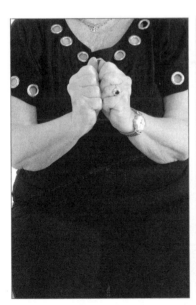 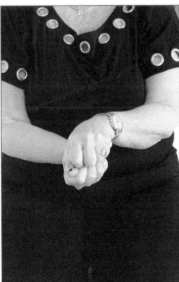 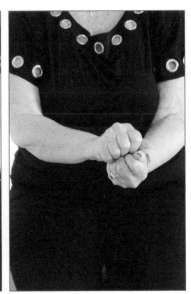

22. Elbow Bends

BENEFITS

This exercise strengthens the muscles that support the elbow and lubricates the corresponding joints.

TECHNIQUE

Sit in any comfortable position. Inhale and extend your arms out in front of you, palms up. Try to keep your shoulders low and relaxed, not scrunched up by your ears. Feel your breath moving up into the higher portion of your lungs. Exhale and touch your fingertips to your shoulders. This is one repetition.

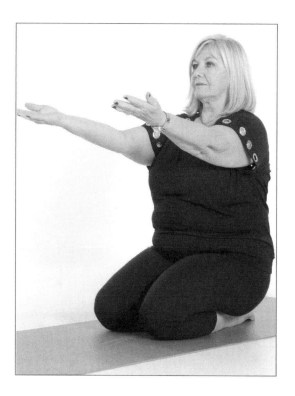 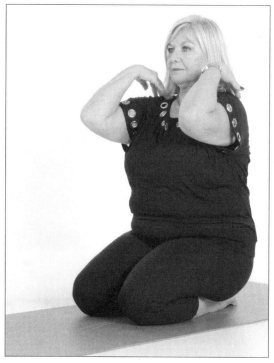

23. Side Stretch

BENEFITS

This exercise stretches your sides, activating muscles that don't get used much when you sit at a desk all day.

TECHNIQUE

Sitting in dandasana or sukhasana (see inset on page 85), inhale and bring your arms out to either side of you. Keep your arms and shoulders soft and relaxed—your fingertips should almost be touching the floor. Exhale and reach your right arm out to the right, creating a stretch on your left side. Inhale and come back to the neutral position. Then exhale and reach your left arm out to the left, creating a stretch on your right side.

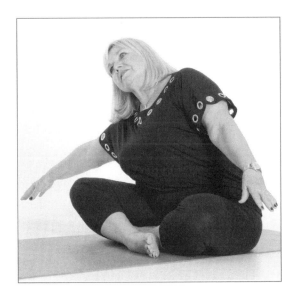
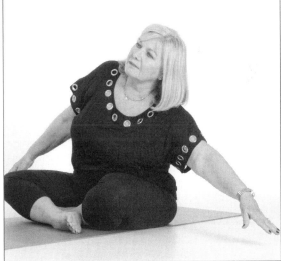

24. Side Twist

BENEFITS

Twists are beneficial to the adrenal glands and organs toward the back of your body, including your kidneys. They also help to relieve and prevent spinal stiffness.

TECHNIQUE

Sit in a comfortable position, such as sukhasana, with your arms out to either side of you, as in the previous exercise. Inhale. Then, as you exhale, twist to your left side. Think of the twist as beginning at the base of the spine and working its way up. Bring your head around to the left side last, keeping your chin parallel to the floor. Inhale and bring your body back to the starting position, leading with your head and unwinding top to bottom. Exhale and continue with a twist to the right side. This is one repetition.

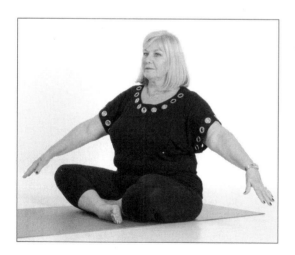 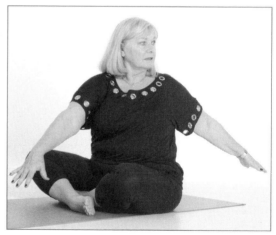

25. Upper Back Opener

BENEFITS

This exercise engages your thoracic vertebrae—the bones in the middle of your spinal column. These vertebrae are critical to moving and bending freely, but are ordinarily difficult to access. Using this exercise will help keep your thoracic vertebrae flexible.

TECHNIQUE

Sitting comfortably in the pose you like best, place your fingertips on top of your shoulders. Inhale and bring your elbows close together in front of your body. Exhale and move your elbows apart, bringing them behind your body as if to make them meet in the middle of your back. (Don't worry, they won't!) Allow your fingertips to remain on top of your shoulders. Feel the squeeze between your shoulder blades.

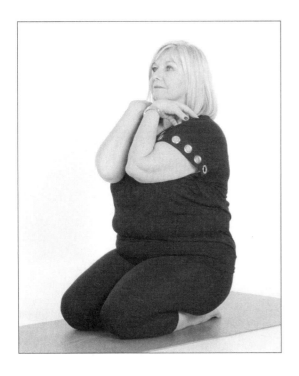 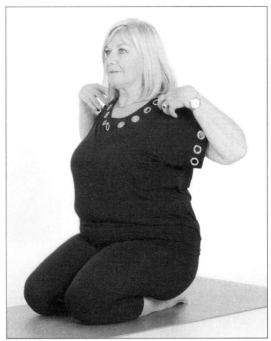

26. Scarecrow

BENEFITS

The scarecrow exercise helps to strengthen the muscles that support your shoulder area. By keeping these muscles strong, you increase your shoulder mobility and prevent rotator cuff injury.

TECHNIQUE

Sitting comfortably in the pose you like best, inhale and bring both arms up and out to your sides, forearms perpendicular to the floor and palms facing forward. Your elbows should be slightly lower than shoulder height. Exhale and rotate your arms at the elbows, bringing your palms down, parallel to the floor.

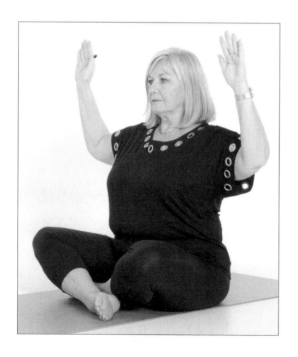 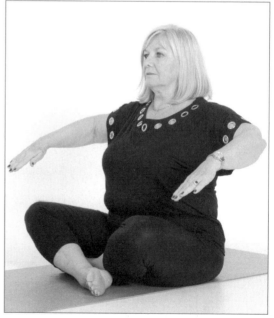

27. Forward & Backward Arch

BENEFITS

This exercise improves mobility in your lower and middle back. Arching your spine forward and backward increases flexibility and rids your joints of foreign substances that may inhibit movement or cause inflammation.

TECHNIQUE

Sitting cross-legged, inhale and take hold of your ankles. Arch your back forward, rotating your shoulders backward and squeezing your shoulder blades toward each other. Your chin will lift slightly, but take care not to scrunch the back of your neck too much. Move your hands to your knees and exhale, arching your body backward, drawing your belly into your spine and tucking your chin into your chest. Notice your shoulder blades opening wide. Return to your starting position. This is one repetition.

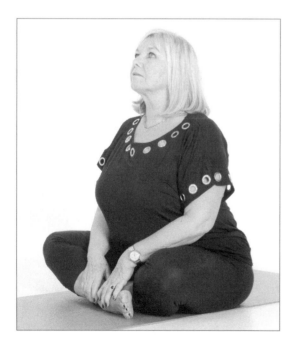
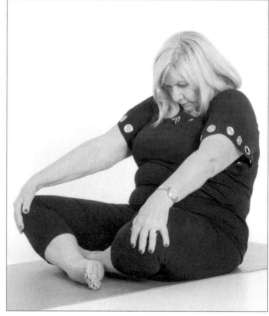

28. Shoulder Lubricator

BENEFITS

This exercise brings tremendous amounts of energy into your body and tones the muscles that allow your shoulder blades to move.

TECHNIQUE

Kneel with your thighs perpendicular to the floor and your weight balanced on your knees and lower legs. If this is uncomfortable, cushion your knees with a folded blanket, or simply sit cross-legged or in vajrasana. Inhale and reach your arms out in front and up overhead, palms facing each other. Don't scrunch up your shoulders; try to keep them relaxed. Exhale and bring your arms down and behind you, palms still facing each other. Notice your shoulder blades squeezing together. If you like, you can add a little "hah!" as your arms come behind your body. This is one repetition.

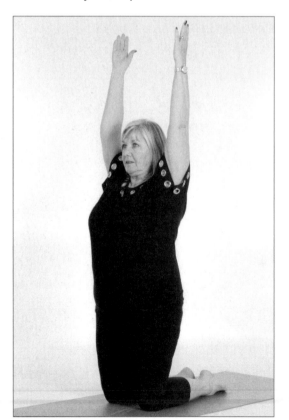

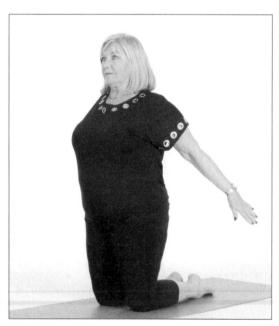

29. Say Yes!

BENEFITS

This exercise increases the mobility of your neck, allowing you to say yes to life!

TECHNIQUE

Sit comfortably in the pose you like best, with your hands placed loosely on top of your knees, palms facing up. Inhale and gently lift your chin. Don't force your chin all the way up—you don't want to jam the back of your neck! Exhale and drop your chin back to your chest. This is one repetition.

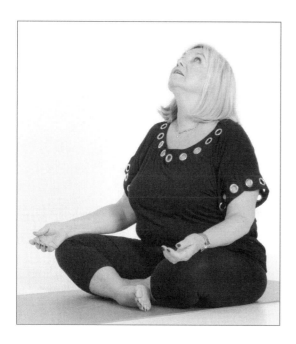
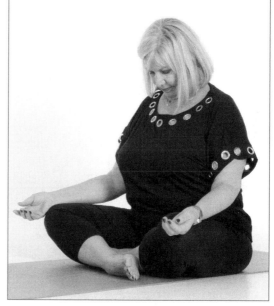

30. Say No!

BENEFITS

This stretch will improve your neck's range of motion and may help you say no to old bad habits.

TECHNIQUE

Sit comfortably in the pose you like best. Inhale and bring your head to a neutral position, facing forward. Exhale and turn your head to the right side, keeping your chin parallel to the floor. Don't go beyond your comfort zone. Inhale and bring your head back to neutral. Then exhale again and turn your head to the left, keeping your chin parallel to the floor. This is one repetition.

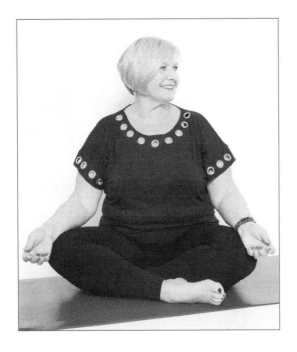 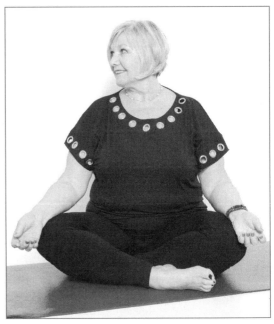

31. Curious Dog

BENEFITS

This exercise also increases your neck's mobility.

TECHNIQUE

Sit comfortably in the pose you like best. If you've been sitting for a long time in one particular pose and are getting less comfortable, change poses! Inhale and bring your hands to rest on your knees or lap. As you exhale, bend your head as if to bring your right ear to your right shoulder. Feel the stretch in the left side of your neck. Inhale and bring your head back to a neutral position. On the next exhale, bend your head to the left, as if to bring your left ear to your left shoulder. Feel the stretch in the right side of your neck. This is one repetition.

Tip: Check yourself by doing this in front of a mirror. You want to make sure that you're not dropping your head or chin forward.

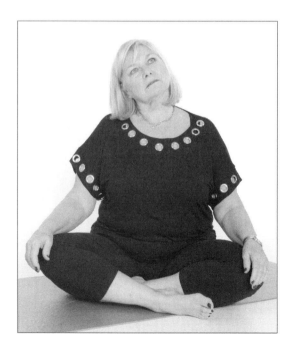
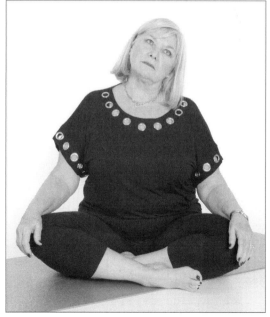

Chapter 6

Breathing Practices

If you've started practicing the physical sequences from the previous chapter, you have already become more aware of your breath, as many of the poses are coordinated with your inhalations and exhalations. In addition to the physical postures, ancient Yogis gave us another tool to combat stress: *pranayama*, or simple breath work. Yogic scriptures first described these breathing practices five thousand years ago, recommending their use as a way to calm and de-fog the mind. The word *pranayama* has two root words: *prana* and *yama*. *Prana* means energy or life force, and is similar to the concept of *chi* or *ki* in Asian philosophies. *Yama* means control. Put them together, and you get *pranayama*, or "energy control."

> "When the breath wanders, the mind also is unsteady. But when the breath is calmed, the mind, too, will be still, and the Yogi achieves long life. Therefore, one should learn to control the breath."
>
> —SWAMI SVATMARAMA, COMPILER OF THE *HATHA YOGA PRADIPIKA*

You see, according to Yogic philosophy, prana is the vital energy that is necessary for any kind of motion. You get this vital energy from many sources, but the most important source is the air. As you breathe, you take in not only oxygen, but prana, which is then distributed throughout your body. Pranayama teaches you how to regulate your breath. By regulating your breath, you regulate your energy, and by extension, your mind. Once you are able to control the prana in your own body and mind, you can begin controlling the universal prana as well. Essentially, you are doing what Yoda told Luke Skywalker to do in *Star Wars*—you are using "the force!"

How does pranayama help relieve stress? Well, on the most basic level, it allows you to refill depleted energy stores. Stress robs you of energy, causing fatigue, depression, and anxiety. It casts a veil over your "inner light," preventing you from accessing your spiritual center. According to Sri Patanjali, compiler of the Yoga Sutras, through pranayama, the "veil over the inner light is destroyed."

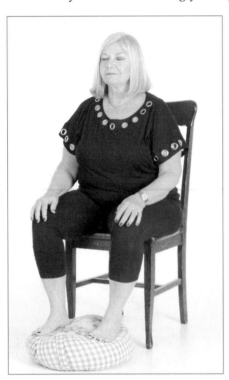

To put it in more practical terms, when you're under pressure, it's almost as if you are leaking energy out of your body—you may even have been aware of this happening to you! I used to teach music to grade-school children, and after a day spent cheerfully singing, dancing, and managing children, I would often come home feeling completely spent. But after a few rounds of nerve purifying breath (see page 106) and a short meditation, I'd feel as good as new. I'd be able to spend the evening doing something fun and creative instead of sitting on the couch and watching TV.

In the exercises that follow, you'll learn a number of different types of pranayama techniques that will allow you to tap into the limitless fund of energy available to us, helping you revitalize or relax. You can practice pranayama after you complete a Yoga pose sequence or before you meditate. You can also practice it separately whenever you feel the need for a little pick-me-up. The more you deepen our breath throughout the day—and you may find yourself doing it automatically after a while— the more energy you'll have. You'll also notice you have better concentration and that you're less likely to get rattled when deadlines loom.

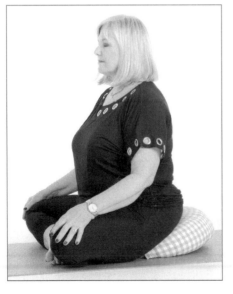

You don't need special props or clothes to practice pranayama, and you can do it in any stable seated position—in a chair or cross-legged on the floor, for example. If you choose to sit in a chair, place a pillow under your feet if they don't naturally reach the floor. If you prefer to sit cross-legged on the floor, use a pillow or zafu under your buttocks to elevate your hips, allowing your legs to open and relax. You can also put pillows under your knees to prop them up for even more comfort.

Breathing Techniques

There are several different breathing techniques in Yoga. Before you learn about them, take a minute to evaluate the way you breathe now. Do you inhale and exhale through your nose or through your mouth? Additionally, observe how your stomach moves when you breathe. Does your stomach move in or out when you inhale? Does it move in or out when you exhale? Most of us are conditioned to hold our stomachs in so that we appear thinner. This leads to "reverse breathing": instead of expanding your belly when you inhale, you're sucking it in, and instead of pulling in your belly when you exhale, you're pushing it out.

In the following techniques, you will be breathing through your nose unless otherwise noted. You will also be breathing from your core, expanding your belly during inhalations and allowing it to contract during exhalations. Essentially, pranayama can help you relearn how to breathe! The rewards are great. Through belly breathing, you'll be able to use your lungs to their full capacity, so that you can take advantage of the wellspring of energy available to us all.

It may take some time for you to get used to this way of breathing, as it goes against what so many of us are used to doing. Try this exercise to train yourself to breathe from your core: Lie on the floor or in bed and place a book on your belly, just below your belly button. Breathe deeply. The book will rise as you inhale—see if you can get it to fall off! It's almost impossible to breathe incorrectly in this position. Continue for five or ten minutes, or for as long as it takes for you to stop reverse breathing automatically. Practice this exercise every day for a week at the beginning of your pranayama practice, and it will soon feel comfortable and natural, as it's the way the body is designed to breathe. You'll soon be ready to begin performing pranayama in a chair or in a comfortable cross-legged position.

Experiment with combining the various breathing practices. It's always good to begin any pranayama session with a few rounds of the simple three-part breath, so that you shift out of shallow breathing and start using a more expansive breath. Then, if your main focus is to calm down, go right into nerve purifying breath. Or, if you are feeling spacey and unfocused, try a few rounds of skull shining breath. Afterwards, if you feel overstimulated, you can balance yourself with a few rounds of nerve purifying breath. The other techniques I offer here can be done as needed, according to the effect you're trying to achieve. For instance, I usually practice the wheezing breath when I'm thirsty or feeling sleepy on the road. The humming bee breath is one I teach at the end of my Hatha Yoga classes. My students enjoy the profound sense of peace that it evokes. I encourage you to try these techniques and notice the effect they have on you!

These are just a few of the many powerful pranayama practices. To learn more techniques, you may want to study with a trained Yoga professional. For your convenience, I've also included some suggestions for books on pranayama in the Resources section at the back of this book.

32. Simple Three-Part Breath
Deergha Swasam

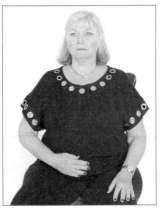

BENEFITS

The simple three-part breath, or *deergha swasam,* is the foundation of all the breathing practices. The "three parts" of the exercise's name are the abdomen, the rib cage/middle chest, and the upper chest. When you do this exercise correctly, you should effectively fill all three of these parts with air, allowing your body to take in up to seven times more air than in normal breathing. More air means more prana—more vitality and more joy!

When you are agitated or upset, this exercise can help calm your mind. Conversely, when you are drowsy or sluggish, the exercise can also perk you up and bring fresh energy into your system. If you have time for only one pranayama practice, this is the one to do. It can be done as a stand-alone practice anytime and anywhere. You can even do it driving in your car or riding on the subway.

TECHNIQUE

Begin by sitting in a comfortable position, either cross-legged on the floor or in a chair with your feet planted about twelve inches apart. Elongate your spine, widen your shoulders, and, unless you're driving or performing another activity that requires your vision, close your eyes softly. Observe your breath.

To perform this exercise, you will be deepening your breath from the bottom up. Place one hand on your lower abdomen. Inhale, expanding your belly as if it were a big balloon. Exhale and empty your lungs, contracting your belly and drawing it up towards your spine to empty your lungs. Throughout, your breaths should be deep, quiet, slow, and controlled. Inhale and exhale a few times to familiarize yourself with the deep belly breath.

Next, move your hand to your lap and put your other hand on the area above your belly button. Inhale and fill both your belly and your rib cage with air, expanding the breath from the bottom

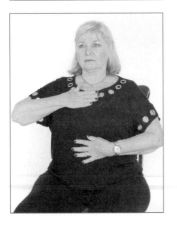

of your lungs on upwards. Exhale slowly, releasing air first from your rib cage, and then from your belly. Repeat a few times.

Finally, move your free hand to your chest, keeping your other hand above your belly button. Inhale and fill first your belly, then your rib cage, and lastly your upper chest with air. You may feel your collarbone rising slightly, but don't let your shoulders creep up. Exhale slowly, emptying your lungs from top to bottom: upper chest first, then rib cage, then belly. You have now completed one round of the simple three-part breath. Once you have an awareness of all three parts, the practice becomes a single continuous flow of breath, in and out. After you get used to the expansion of the abdomen, rib cage, and upper chest, allow your hands to come to rest on your lap—they're only there to guide you as you're learning to sense what it feels like to breathe deeply.

The calming effect of the three-part breath comes from generating deep belly breaths and long, slow exhalations. If your breathing is quick and agitated at first, it may take a bit of concentration to control and slow it down. When you're upset, you usually breathe from the upper chest. It may help to inhale deeply and then exhale forcefully through your mouth—saying "ha!" loudly as you do so—to prepare you for the slower, quieter breathing this exercise requires. Do this a few times, imagining that each time you exhale, you are releasing anxiety through your breath. Then begin the calmer three-part breath.

DURATION

Beginner: Start by focusing only on filling your belly, allowing it to puff out a bit. Build your breath by gradually starting to fill your rib cage and upper chest. As a standalone practice, the three-part breath can be practiced for long periods of time—anywhere from three to fifteen minutes. As preparation for one of the other meditations offered later in this chapter, three to five minutes should be sufficient.

Intermediate: When you are comfortable with the full lung expansion, you can begin to count and compare inhalations to exhalations. If, without straining, you are able to control your exhalations so that they are at least as long as your inhalations, begin to extend your exhalations so that they are as much as twice as long as your inhalations. For better control, use *ujjayi,* the hissing breath, as seen on page 110. When your exhalations are longer than your inhalations, relaxation is virtually guaranteed!

CONSIDERATIONS

Be sure to monitor the movement of your abdomen. If you find you are pulling in your belly on the inhalation, you are doing what we call "reverse breathing." To avoid reverse breathing, try the exercise discussed on page 101.

33. Skull Shining Breath
Kapalabhati

BENEFITS

Also known as the "breath of fire," the skull shining breath helps clear and purify the skull's *nadis,* or energy channels, refreshing the brain. Because of its heating properties, it also energizes the body and removes impurities in the bloodstream. It can be especially useful to perform the skull shining breath in the afternoon, when you might ordinarily have reached for a cup of coffee or a cocktail.

TECHNIQUE

Sit comfortably, with your spine long and your shoulders wide. Do two or three rounds of the three-part breath. After the last exhalation, draw a short inhalation, filling only your belly with air. Then, with a snap of the abdomen, pull your belly in towards your spine and force your breath out through your nostrils, as if you are trying to blow a feather off the tip of your nose. This exhalation requires the same force used to blow your nose, so be sure to have a tissue handy just in case! Continue with short inhalations into your belly and quick, forceful exhalations. After the last round, finish with a full three-part inhalation and a long, slow exhalation.

DURATION

Beginner: I recommend performing three rounds of ten to twenty repetitions.

Intermediate: You can increase the number of repetitions per round to between sixty and eighty—as many as you can complete without straining yourself. If you are taking Yoga classes regularly, you may be encouraged to hold your breath at the end of the final inhalation; please do this only under the guidance of a seasoned Yoga teacher.

CONSIDERATIONS

If you begin to feel dizzy, please stop and take a break. You can try again later if you wish, but don't overdo it. You don't want to hyperventilate! The shining skull breath is not recommended for women who are menstruating, pregnant, or postpartum. Those with high blood pressure or other forms of heart disease, lung disease such as asthma, or ulcers or hernias, should not perform this exercise without the guidance of a seasoned Yoga teacher. In addition, I do not recommend this exercise for people who use recreational drugs or alcohol to excess. Because of its capacity to stimulate, the skull shining breath can overwhelm a person whose nervous system may already be compromised by the debilitating effects of toxic substances.

This is a very invigorating practice and should be followed by a more calming breath, such as the one on the next page.

34. Nerve Purifying Breath

Nadi suddhi

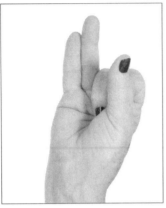

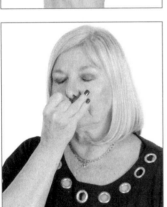

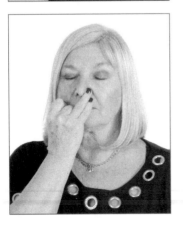

BENEFITS

Nadi suddhi, the nerve purifying breath or alternate nostril breath, is, with the simple three-part breath and the skull shining breath, one of the three primary breathing practices that are all ideally performed at the end of a physical posture sequence. It's also effective to help calm the mind right before a meditation session.

Nerve purifying breath is a gentle technique that balances the right and left brain and has a relaxing effect on the mind. It helps to alleviate stress by harmonizing the totality of prana in the body. It may also alleviate hypertension, as the practice stimulates various nerves that reach different areas of the hypothalamus, a part of the brain that helps regulate blood pressure.

TECHNIQUE

Sit comfortably, with your spine long and your shoulders wide. After getting settled in your comfortable posture, you will use your right hand to make a gesture known as *Vishnu mudra*—a sacred hand position associated with Vishnu, the Hindu god known as the preserver of the universe. To do this mudra, make a gentle fist and then extend your thumb, pinky, and ring finger. Tuck your right elbow close to your chest and bring your thumb close to your right nostril. Inhale through both nostrils, then block off your right nostril with your thumb as you exhale out of the left nostril, using the simple three-part breath (see page 102). Inhale through your left nostril and then block it off with your extended pinky and ring finger, removing your thumb from your right nostril so that you can exhale from it. Inhale right, exhale left. Continue in this pattern, switching nostrils after each inhalation. Finish with an exhalation out of your right nostril. Bring your hands to your lap and take a moment to feel the peaceful effect of this practice.

DURATION

Beginner: Practice the alternate nostril breath for up to three minutes.

Intermediate: If you're comfortable with this practice, you can extend the duration up to fifteen minutes, being careful not to strain. Compare the length of your inhalations and exhalations, and gradually work up to having your exhalations be twice as long as your inhalations. For example: inhale to the count of five, and exhale to the count of ten. You can count using simple numbers, or, to help you space your breaths more evenly, you can add "om" or "peace" in between the numbers: "Om one. . .om two. . .om three. . .om four. . .om five. . ." In Yoga, we spiritualize everything!

CONSIDERATIONS

Do not strain as you lengthen your exhalations. Keep your breath soft and fluid each time you switch nostrils. Although these breathing techniques have been shown to lower blood pressure, you should not forego medication or conventional treatment for hypertension without first consulting your doctor.

35. Wheezing Breath
Sitkari

BENEFIT

This breath cools the body, purifies and stimulates the gums, and also helps wake you up if you're sleepy. In addition, it may quench your thirst and even assuage hunger! I use it during the fall allergy season, when my nose gets stuffed up and my regular pranayama practices are difficult to do. It's helpful as a stress management tool because it brings your awareness back to your breathing, increases prana in the system, and cleans the nadis. It also helps to cool excited emotions and relieve mental tensions.

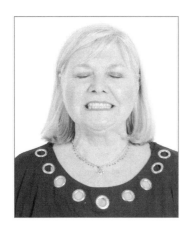

TECHNIQUE

Sit comfortably, with your spine long and your shoulders wide. Close your eyes and become aware of your breath, allowing it to slow down and become more rhythmic. After a minute or two, bare your teeth and curl your tongue back so that it touches the soft palate on the roof of your mouth. You should look like you're wearing a wide, maniacal grin. Inhale through your teeth, making a wet, slurpy sound. You will feel a coolness as the air enters the sides of your mouth. Hold the breath for a few seconds, close your mouth, and then exhale slowly out of your nostrils.

DURATION

Beginner: Try three repetitions.

Intermediate: Try five to eight repetitions. If you find that the exercise overstimulates you, follow with the nerve purifying breath to calm you down.

CONSIDERATIONS

Do not perform the wheezing breath in very cold weather or in a heavily polluted environment. It's also not recommended for those with untreated low blood pressure, asthma, or bronchitis.

36. Humming Bee Breath
Bhramari

BENEFITS

The humming bee breath provides a real experience of bliss by having you mimic the primordial hum of the universe—a vibration that is the life force that is present in everything and everybody. It is a soothing practice, ideal for promoting sleep and alleviating depression. It strengthens the voice and eliminates throat ailments, and has been proven to speed up healing. The humming bee breath can be used instead of the nerve purifying breath as a preparation for meditation. It's also just fun to do!

TECHNIQUE

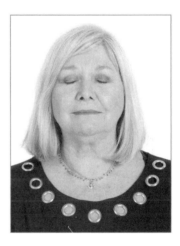

Sit comfortably, with your spine long and your shoulders wide. Close your eyes and do two or three rounds of the simple three-part breath. When you are ready, inhale deeply through the nostrils and, with your teeth slightly separated and lips gently closed, begin humming as you exhale. Continue to hum, smoothly and evenly, at any pitch, until all the air is expelled. Observe the pleasant buzzing in your head and imagine the vibrations going straight up through the crown of your head and out into the universe. When you run out of breath, you have completed one round and can inhale again. Allow your mind to become absorbed by the humming sound.

DURATION

Do five rounds of the humming bee breath, at various pitches, without opening your eyes. Once you've finished, sit quietly and listen. You should hear the humming continuing inside you. As you become better attuned to this subtle humming, which is called *pranava,* you'll begin to realize that it goes on all the time! Awareness of pranava can help you access the deep peace of your true nature.

37. Hissing Breath
Ujjayi

BENEFITS

In Yogic breathing, the longer you are able to exhale, the greater the benefits to your system. A slow exhalation helps your body distribute prana into the most subtle areas of the body—the cells, and even the spaces between the cells! One way to prolong your exhalations is through the hissing breath, or *ujjayi.* This practice helps calm your mind and focus restless thoughts. It also increases circulation to your throat and improves digestion and respiratory problems.

TECHNIQUE

Sit comfortably, with your spine long and your shoulders wide. Begin by closing your eyes and mouth and relaxing your entire body. Take some time to watch your breath, allowing it to gradually slow down and become more rhythmic. Inhale, bringing your awareness to your throat, and as you exhale slowly, partially contract the glottis muscles at the back of your throat. This will create a gentle hissing sound, so subtle that only you will be able to hear it. It's the same sound that a sleeping baby makes, almost like a soft snore. Another way to ensure that you are doing ujjayi correctly is to first open your mouth and hiss like an angry cat. Now try the same hiss, closing your mouth and your glottis. After you have inhaled and exhaled once in this manner, you have completed a round.

DURATION

Beginner: This exercise is not recommended for beginners.

Intermediate: Do up to eight rounds. As you become comfortable with this exercise, try to make your exhalations twice as long as your inhalations.

CONSIDERATIONS

This exercise is not recommended for beginners. Avoid straining your throat by slowly building up to a longer practice over time.

Chapter 7

Meditation Practices

Meditation is yet another method we can use to reduce the stress in our lives. In this chapter, you'll find descriptions and photographs of various meditation techniques that you can easily incorporate into your daily routine. Some techniques are relaxing and will help to calm you down, but I've also included a few techniques that are stimulating and will help to improve your mood when you're feeling depressed.

"The well-trained mind of a yogi, concentrating on the Self, is as steady as a flame in a windless place."
—BHAGAVAD GITA 6:19

These meditations are not sequential. Instead, they are divided into four categories, each focusing on a specific cause of stress: grief or loss, problems with loved ones, illness or injury, and money trouble. This allows you to find the meditation that is best suited to your situation. You shouldn't feel limited to the section that addresses your particular problem, though; a meditation from the section on grief may be just as effective when used to alleviate stress from financial woes, for example. There are no rules here.

It may take time for you to get comfortable with meditation, especially if you're new to the practice. You may initially feel you're doing it wrong. My advice is this: don't judge your experience. There is no "right" way to meditate. If a certain meditation feels good, continue practicing it. If you get restless with one approach, try another approach the next time you sit down for meditation. Mix and match meditations until you find a meditation or combination of meditations that brings you deep into your inner peace and contentment.

And keep at it. Sri Patanjali tells us that we will succeed in meditation when we "practice for a long time, without break, and in all earnestness." Try not to worry about the results. Even experienced meditators have a dud from time to time! Meditation is a personal practice; it's all about finding the approach that works best for you, sticking with it, and doing it regularly. Remember, you will get significant benefits just by giving yourself the opportunity to slow down, take a few deep breaths, and watch your mind. It may sound daunting, but you will notice an improvement after even one session, so imagine how much it will help if you meditate more often.

Before we get started, let's take a closer look at meditation—what it is, what its benefits are, and how you should begin your practice.

WHAT IS MEDITATION?

Meditation is a process by which you bring your mind into focus over a long and uninterrupted period of time. This can be exceptionally useful for those of us whose minds are filled with chatter—thoughts about obligations, needs, emotions, conversations, social interactions, and all the other daily concerns. All these competing thoughts can make us feel overburdened and stressed out! Through meditation, you learn how to quiet this incessant flow of thought and regain a sense of peace and tranquility.

Meditation involves two of the eight important disciplines or practices that, according to the sage Patanjali, all Yogis need to practice in order to gain mastery over the mind, body, and senses. As described by Patanjali in the Yoga Sutras, these eight disciplines and practices can be seen as branches of a tree, all contributing equally to the health and well-being of the tree's core. You've already learned about two of the other limbs—the physical poses (*asana*, the third branch) and breath work (*pranayama*, the fourth branch). Meditation as we understand it today encompasses both the sixth limb of the tree—*dharana*, or "concentration,"—and the seventh limb of the tree—*dhyana*, or "true meditation."

Dharana is what people usually have in mind when they think of meditation. In it, you concentrate on a chosen object of meditation and direct your mind back to this object whenever your mind wanders. Dhyana occurs when you are able to train a continuous flow of thought onto one point. As you become more adept at dharana, you will find that dhyana occurs spontaneously.

When you meditate, you automatically begin practicing the fifth of the eight practices: *pratyahara,* or withdrawal of the senses. In pratyahara, you turn your senses away from external stimuli (the phone ringing, the smell of dinner being cooked, etc.), and focus on your inner experience. Essentially, you pull back into yourself, like a turtle retreating into its shell. There are many different ways to withdraw your senses. Closing your eyes is the most obvious—you put your sense of sight on hold, so that whatever might come into view will not distract you. Without these distractions, your mind becomes clear and calm, perfectly ready for meditation!

And finally, once you have mastered both dharana and dhyana, you may be able to attain *samadhi,* the eighth and final practice Patanjali described. Samadhi

The Eight-Limbed Tree of Yoga

According to the sage Patanjali, there are eight disciplines and practices that every would-be Yogi should master in order to attain better control over the mind. These "limbs" include:

1. *Yama.* This concept, loosely translated as "self-restraint," informs five ethical principles to be observed in dealing with the external world: practice nonviolence and respect for all living things, be truthful in word and deed, refrain from theft or coveting, practice sexual abstinence and moderation in all things, and refrain from greediness and hoarding.

2. *Niyama.* Niyama, or "observance," is a companion concept to yama; it informs five principles that apply to your personal life. Niyama asks that you practice purity (cleanliness of body and mind), contentment, austerity, spiritual study and self-examination, and surrender (devotion to a higher power).

3. *Asana.* The physical poses of Yoga, some of which you learned in Chapter 5. Yogis believe that it is difficult to control the mind without also being able to control the body.

4. *Pranayama.* Energy control through breathing practices, as discussed in Chapter 6.

5. *Pratyahara.* This term, which means "withdrawal of the senses," refers to the practice of drawing your focus away from the outside world and inward to the radiant peace and bliss of your own true nature.

6. *Dharana.* Dharana, or "concentration," is what most people have in mind when they think of meditation. It is the process by which you fixate on a specific object in order to sharpen your focus and control and calm your mind.

7. *Dhyana.* Dhyana means "meditation," or the ability to direct and maintain a continuous stream of thoughts onto a single object. It occurs naturally as a refinement of dharana—that is, as you become more skilled at dharana, you will be able to attain dhyana almost as a matter of course.

8. *Samadhi.* Samadhi, understood as "self-realization" or "liberation," is the most advanced level of Yoga—an elevated state of consciousness that represents unity with the infinite consciousness.

can be understood as "liberation" or "self-realization." It is a state of higher consciousness, an experience of bliss that comes of being at one with the universe and the divine. According to spiritual master Sri Chinmoy, in the state of samadhi, ". . .you enjoy a supremely divine, all-pervading, self-amorous ecstasy. You become the object of enjoyment, you become the enjoyer, and you become the enjoyment itself." Through samadhi, one can achieve moksha, or liberation.

BENEFITS OF MEDITATION

Meditation has many benefits, both for your health in general and for the alleviation of a wide range of more specific stress-related health challenges. It should come as no surprise that meditation has great advantages for your mental state. Concentration, productivity, memory, and mood all improve with regular meditation practice. According to some scientists, this is because frequent meditation creates long-lasting changes in the structure, adaptability, and electrical activity of the brain. In particular, research has shown that meditation stimulates activity in the left prefrontal cortex, an area of the brain associated with happiness and better energy levels; it simultaneously decreases activity in the amygdala, your emotional center, and your right prefrontal cortex, an area associated with anxiety and stress. One study found that depressed patients who practiced meditation as part of their recovery process were 50 percent less likely to relapse. Meditation can also be a powerful tool for ending or curbing addictions; it reduces the anxieties and other mental disturbances that can lead to substance abuse and teaches people to react more calmly to emotionally arousing stimuli.

"An inspired mind has power."
—SWAMI RAMANANDA

Perhaps most surprising, some studies indicate that regular meditation also increases the thickness of brain regions connected to attention, memory, decision-making, and sensory processing. This allows for enhanced functioning—a higher capacity noted in one study of middle-school students, who saw improvements in attendance, grade point average, and work habits after learning to meditate consistently.

But the benefits of meditation aren't limited to the mind. In one study, inner-city residents with symptoms of anxiety, depression, diabetes, or hypertension saw a 50 percent reduction in psychiatric symptoms, a 70 percent reduction in anxiety, and a 44 percent reduction in medical problems. Scientists hypothesize that meditation boosts the natural immune response, making regular meditators more resistant to illness and disease. Research bears this out—one health insurance study found that meditators took half as many visits to the doctor as did nonmeditators. In addition, meditators had 87 percent fewer hospitalizations. Meditation has been shown to reduce high blood pressure, blood sugar levels, heart disease, chronic pain, and other serious conditions. Moreover, the immune system boost seemed to last for a time even after patients stopped meditating.

Finally, meditation has profound implications for the aging process. According to the National Center for Complementary and Integrative Health, a branch of the National Institutes of Health, regular meditation can actually improve longevity and quality of life. People who meditate often look younger than they really are!

It's amazing that the benefits of this ancient practice can now be studied and quantified by our modern technologies. With all this convincing evidence on the advantages of meditation, I know you'll want to get right into it.

PREPARING FOR MEDITATION

In preparing to meditate, the first thing you'll need to do is to find a comfortable seat, since you'll be sitting very still for a while. Try sitting cross-legged on the floor, using a pillow under your buttocks. If you like, you can buy a zafu, as described earlier. Or you might want to try a slanted meditation bench. If you don't want to sit on the floor, you can sit in a straight-backed chair instead, taking care to keep your spine long and your shoulders wide—a position that allows energy to flow upward to your higher energy centers. No matter how you choose to sit, the key is to find a comfortable position that you'll be able to maintain for the duration of your meditation. Make a vow, or *sankalpa*, that you are not going to move a muscle until you finish.

Meditation can be performed as a standalone session, or it can be combined with any of the other practices discussed in this book. In my Yoga classes, I like to start with a centering chant or prayer, continue with a sequence of physical poses, guided relaxation, and pranayama, and then finish with a short meditation. This order allows you to progressively and systematically move from the physical—your body—to the metaphysical/spiritual—your breath and mind. As you'll see, the results can be profoundly relaxing. Still, not everybody has time to do Yoga poses *and* breathing practices *and* meditation. In that case, listen to my teacher, who said that if you have time for nothing else, you should at least sit for meditation. If you can carve out half an hour to meditate, great! But even a brief session can be immensely helpful.

When should you meditate? The best time to meditate is at dawn, before your mind gets cluttered with all the events and obligations of the day. If you have a hard time waking up early and find yourself dozing during meditation, try doing a few stretches from any of the sequences found in Chapter 5 before you start. You might try splashing some cold water on your face, taking a cool shower, or having a cup of tea to make your mind more alert. It can also be helpful to meditate before bedtime, as meditation helps calm your mind so you can have a good night's sleep. But really, you should meditate at whatever time is convenient for you. Routine meditation at a time that fits into your schedule is better than sporadic practice at dawn.

When you begin to meditate, try to sit for ten or fifteen minutes twice a day. As you become more comfortable with your practice, you can gradually extend the length of your sessions. That said, it's better to meditate for two short periods every day than to meditate for an hour once a week. The keys are to tend to the process of meditation, not the goal—and to practice meditation regularly.

Putting Your Yoga Practices Together

Don't let your stress management routine give you more stress! One of the major advantages of Big Yoga is that it is very flexible and can easily be adapted to fit into your busy schedule. I recommend that you try to do a little something every day—just five minutes of meditation can make a big difference when it comes to your stress levels! But don't worry if you've having trouble making the time to do asanas, pranayama, and meditation every day. Instead, add, subtract, and pair practices according to your needs and preferences. For instance, if you're stuck on a plane, you could do the seated sequence and then go into a few minutes of pranayama. Or, if you're at work and you need to get up and move around, do the salute to the sun and follow it with a quick body scan. And if you prefer meditation to pranayama, by all means, spend more time meditating!

At home, I recommend that you set aside a whole hour for self-care once a week. Ideally, in that hour, you would do the Flex-Ability series and then continue with deep relaxation, pranayama, and meditation—in that sequence. As I explained on page 115, I find it most relaxing to shift focus from the body (asanas) to the breath (pranayama) to the mind (meditation). Even if you can't do all three, I recommend following this basic order: asanas before pranayama, pranayama before meditation. If you don't have time for a full hour, try just ten minutes of pranayama, followed by five minutes of meditation. Or do Yoga Nidra and then some chanting. You get the idea—mix it up. Keep trying new combinations, changing and adjusting your routines as you see fit. The key is to do whatever works for you in order to integrate Yoga practices into your life. Even a little bit of Yoga can make a big difference.

38. So-Hum Meditation
Ajapa japa

BENEFITS

The ancient so-hum meditation is the easiest and most basic one you'll learn. If you try the so-hum meditation and enjoy it, you may not need to read any further—that's how effective it is. In the so-hum meditation, you focus on your breath as it enters and leaves your body. This meditation calms the mind, is helpful for insomnia and heart disease, and creates inner stability. Best of all, the so-hum meditation can be done any- where! You can do it in a formal meditation session, or you can simply listen to your breath when you're on the subway, stuck in traffic, or taking a walk. As you focus on the breath, you will find yourself entering a deeper state of relaxation. Enjoy that!

> *"Meditation is the ultimate psychology, the ultimate therapy for Mankind."*
> —GOSWAMI KRIYANANDA

TECHNIQUE

In a comfortable seated position, begin by doing a few rounds of the simple three-part breath (see page 102). Then, relax your breath, allowing it to come back to normal, and begin to observe it. As you inhale, notice your belly expanding, and as you exhale, notice your belly collapsing. Feel the sensation of your breath traveling in and out of your nostrils. As it comes in, your breath feels cool. As it leaves, it feels warm. Now notice the speed of your breaths—are your breaths steady? Unsteady? It's all good. Listen to the sound it makes. Can you hear "so" on the inhale, and "hum" on the exhale? These sounds combine to give this exercise its name, which means "I am He" in Sanskrit. "He" is the Universal Self, known as Brahman—in other words, this phrase means that you are no longer the limited self, the little "me." As you hear this mantra, engage your emotions. Feel that you are one with the all-pervading consciousness. This extra bit of devotional oomph will maximize the benefits of this calming meditation.

Don't worry if your mind wanders off and you find yourself thinking about lunch or the laundry. This is a natural part of the process of training your mind. Just bring your attention gently back to the sound and experience of your breaths. Every time you notice that you lost your focus, it's a victory!

This meditation can be enhanced by using ujjayi, the hissing breath described on page 110. To add ujjayi, simply contract the glottis gently during inhalation and exhalation. Ujjayi helps make the breath more audible, raising your awareness of the so-hum meditation.

DURATION

Start with regular fifteen-minute meditations, performed once or twice a day. As you get more comfortable, lengthen your practice to thirty minutes. Gradually, your breaths will become slower as you go deep into your meditation. The repetition of the mantra will fade away as your mind becomes still.

Meditations for Grief

The loss of a loved is always devastating, and can have a significant impact on your health. In 1967, two psychiatrists, Thomas Holmes and Richard Rahe, conducted research to find out how and to what extent stressful events cause serious illness. According to their findings, the death of a spouse had the greatest capacity of all life occurrences to put a person at risk of sickness; the death of other close family members or friends scored slightly lower.

When you lose someone, the hard part comes after the flurry of visits, sympathy cards, and phone calls is over, and you have to try to go back to a normal life. There is no normal life after your child, your lover, your mother, or your father dies. To be fair, there really isn't anything a person can say to somebody who has lost a loved one. This is why we end up repeating platitudes such as "I'm so sorry for your loss." At Yogaville, a swami told me that we're connected to our dearest loved ones with what she described as strings of love. These strings slowly unravel and dissolve when we are separated by death, and that process can be physically painful.

"In the midst of winter, I finally learned that there was, within me, an invincible summer."
—ALBERT CAMUS

But I'll share with you some advice. When a close family member died—Caroline's death was sudden, and shocking—my friend Robin told me this: "Do your grieving right away. Don't wait, don't try to put it off, do it now." And I did. I cried and cried. I cried while I was taking care of my two small children. I cried on the table waiting for the chiropractor to try to get my spine back in the right place. I cried as I wrote in my journal. I had never had anything in my life hit me so hard. Caroline was my big sis—she was the one I trailed behind, the one I looked to, my favorite playmate. I watched her to see how I was supposed to live my life. It took at least a year or so before I was able to get back to normal.

It's important to grieve. But it's also important to move on. You still have to feed the kids, do the dishes, go to work, be a good spouse, and try to make do. Be kind to yourself. One of the sympathy cards I received after my son Sam's death said, "Rest when you're weary," and that really touched me. Grieving can be tiring. You are wounded, so let your spirit heal.

Meditation can help. We are never more in need of something calming as when a loved one has left this earthly plane. A simple meditation session or two each day can make you feel better. In this section, I'll share with you some simple meditations that I found particularly useful throughout the long process of letting go.

Choosing a Mantra

A mantra can come from the sacred words or prayers of any faith or religion, or it can be a nondenominational spiritual affirmation, such as "All is one" or "Love is eternal." Choose a mantra that is comforting to you—shorter mantras are more powerful than longer ones. I find the Sanskrit mantra *om shanti* to be especially helpful, as the word "shanti" not only means peace, but also evokes and embodies the nature of peace. (For more information, see page 142.) As it says in the Bible, "Speak the word only, and I shall be healed."

Besides om shanti, there are many other mantras from various traditions and cultures that you can use. You don't need to belong to a specific religion in order to adopt its mantras! Any sacred words will give you great, calming benefits. Here are a couple of my favorites.

The Gayatri mantra is one of the most ancient mantras, coming from the Rig Veda. It goes:

Om bhur bhuva swaha

Tat savitur varenyam

Bhargo devasya dhimahi

Dhyo yo nah prachodayaat

Roughly translated, this means: We meditate on the glory of that Being who produced this universe; may He enlighten our minds.

The Hare Krishna mantra is a *maha* (great) mantra that celebrates Lord Krishna

and Lord Rama, two divine beings in Hindu mythology. In addition to bestowing peace and happiness, this mantra is said to promote liberation from the cycles of birth and death. Here it is:

Hare Krishna Hare Krishna

Krishna Krishna Hare Hare

Hare Rama Hare Rama

Rama Rama Hare Hare

There are also a number of shorter mantras that you can use. From the Hindu tradition, *hari om* is a mantra that, when chanted aloud, moves energy from the solar plexus (*ha*) up through the center of the body (*ri*) and out through the top of the head at the crown chakra (*om*). From the Tibetan Buddhist tradition, we get the mantra *om mani padme hum,* which translates to "Praises to the jewel in the Lotus," a salutation to the inner teacher that resides in your heart. From the Sikh tradition, there's the mantra *wahe guru, wahe guru, wahe guru jeeo,* which translates to, "The ecstasy of consciousness is my beloved." From the Islamic tradition, try the mantra *allahu akbar,* which means "God is great"; from the Jewish tradition, there's the similar phrase *adonai echad,* which means "The lord our God is one."

Every religion has its own words of power. Choose the mantra that resonates with you—the words should feel good when you repeat them out loud.

39. Mantra Meditation

Mantra Japa

BENEFITS

You may have heard it said that the mind is like a drunken monkey that's been bitten by a scorpion, jumping around from one thing to another. When you're mourning the loss of a loved one, your mind tends to fixate on the past—on mistakes that were made, on anger at the loved one for leaving, and on anxiety about a future that looks frightening without your loved one. A *mantra* can be a soothing balm that heals your wounded heart as it erases negativity from your mind. A mantra is a sacred sound formula, revealed to the ancient seers (*rishis*) in deep meditation. Words like "om," "amen," "alleluia," and "Allah" are all mantras from various cultures and traditions, each one having its own particular flavor and effect on the mind. The Lord's Prayer and the Hail Mary can be considered examples of long-form mantras. *Japa* means repetition. Put the two words together—*mantra japa*—and you have one of the most basic forms of meditation: the repetition of a mantra. You can repeat your mantra anywhere and at any time; your mantra is always with you.

TECHNIQUE

Sitting comfortably, eyes closed, do a few rounds of the simple three-part breath. If you like, you can say an introductory prayer to invoke the presence of the divine, and to give your mind the idea that this is the time to go within. You can use anything—the Lord's Prayer is good, as are the prayers in the inset on page 120. After you've finished your centering prayer, begin your silent mantra repetitions. If your mind is jumpy, you can say the mantra out loud, gradually decreasing your volume, getting softer and softer until your lips are moving without any sound. Then stop moving your lips and silently continue your mantra repetitions. At the end of your meditation, send out positive, loving thoughts to those you have lost, and feel gratitude for their presence, however brief, in your life.

DURATION

Prepare by doing about five minutes of the three-part breath (page 102). Then do your mantra repetition for ten to twenty minutes.

ADAPTATION

If you find that your mind is wandering excessively, you can add the use of a mala, or rosary. For more information, see page 27.

Prayers and Blessings

Many people find it useful to begin their meditation sessions with a prayer. Prayers focus your mind, thus helping you prepare for meditation. Here are two prayers I like to use:

Beloved God, please allow me to worship you here as the mantra. Bless me to feel your presence, and comfort me in my grief.

Salutations to the Supreme God of Love. You know all my problems and sorrows even before I ask for your help, but I humbly ask for your healing blessings, now and always.

Your prayer does not need to address a divine being. If you'd prefer to use a nontheistic prayer, you can instead set a goal or an intention, such as "Nothing will distract me from my meditation," or "My meditation will bring me greater peace of mind, making me fit for service." The idea here is just to get yourself into the right mood for your session.

If you like, you can also end your meditation with a simple blessing, offering the benefits of your practice to the greater good. Just as a prayer can help take you out of your busy day, a blessing gives your mind the signal that you're ready to go back into everyday consciousness. I like to conclude my sessions with these humble but powerful words taken from an ancient Sanskrit saying: "May the entire creation be filled with peace and joy, love and light." But you can use anything you like!

40. Gazing Meditation

Tratak

BENEFIT

My guru encouraged his disciples never to suppress emotion. Instead, he told us to "taste" our tears. The gazing meditation known as *tratak* allows you to do just that, bathing your eyes and rejuvenating them. Recent studies have determined that tears of sadness have a different chemical makeup from tears brought on by chopping an onion. This indicates that emotional tears might have a separate and beneficial purpose in alleviating stress.

In addition, the gazing meditation helps focus your mind when you're feeling scattered.

TECHNIQUE

Sit in front of a candle with the flame at about eye level, six to twelve inches away. Gaze at the flame without blinking and without moving your eyes or head. After a while, you'll experience a slight burning sensation in your eyes; you may even tear up. Keep your eyes open for as long as you can. When you're ready, close your eyes gently, and observe the image of the flame in your mind's eye until it fades away. Open your eyes, gaze at the flame again, and repeat.

If you find yourself beginning to cry, just let it happen. Allow emotions to surface, and witness them without judgment. When those feelings subside, go back to gazing at the flame and continue your practice.

DURATION

Do this technique for five to ten minutes. Then, with your eyes closed, sit quietly for as long as half an hour afterward, observing the effects of this practice.

ADAPTATION

If you prefer, you can fixate on a flower, a crystal, or a picture of a saint or spiritual teacher who inspires you. Alternatively, use a sacred image such as a cross, a *yantra* (mystical diagram), or a *mandala* (spiritual symbol). These iconic images have a special geometry that is said to embody mystical properties. Simply find a point on the image you are using, and steady your gaze. You can even imagine you are imbibing the holy qualities of the image, filling the emptiness you may feel as a result of your devastating loss.

Sacred Geometry

The geometries found in mandalas, crystals, pyramids and labyrinths are essential to understanding the way the universe is designed. Human attention is intuitively drawn to the sacred shapes found in stained-glass windows, Islamic mosaics, Celtic symbols—even the patterns of Sufi dancing. It's as if the meaning of these circles, triangles, and squares is embedded in our DNA. As you meditate on these iconic forms, your concentration gathers strength, bringing you into harmony with the peace and *sat* (truth) of the universe.

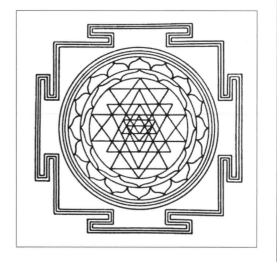

41. Walking Meditation

BENEFITS

Sometimes you just aren't capable of settling down for a formal sitting meditation. At times like these, you might want to consider this walking meditation from the Buddhist tradition. Done slowly, the meditation can be very calming; practiced at a faster and more rhythmic pace, the meditation can help channel any strong emotions. When performed outside, you get the added benefit of connecting with nature.

As you dedicate your attention to your walking, you become more mindful of a process that you perform unthinkingly as part of everyday life. A walking meditation can allow you to feel the connection between your meditations and your daily routines, training your mind to be more present and aware, more often.

TECHNIQUE

Find an unobstructed pathway that's thirty or forty feet long. With your eyes gazing down toward the earth, and your awareness within, slowly walk the length of your pathway. Then turn around and walk back. Continue walking back and forth in this manner, trying not to look at anything in particular. Focus your attention on the rhythm of your movement. Observe the sensations of your feet as they lift, move, and set back down on the ground. To end your meditation, you may want to offer a prayer, such as "May the whole creation be filled with peace and happiness."

DURATION

I recommend that you walk for ten to twenty-five minutes.

ADAPTATIONS

If your mind wanders, you can silently repeat a calming phrase or mantra to the rhythm of your steps in order to help maintain your focus. You may also find it helpful to carry mala beads (see page 27) to enhance your concentration.

Meditations for Problems with Loved Ones

We all have to work to maintain good relationships with our loved ones, whether they are family, friends, or romantic partners. The people who matter most can bring out the best in us, but they can also bring out the worst, resulting in anger, frustration, and sorrow. We snap at our children when they don't clean their rooms, exchange sharp words with our spouses when they forget to run important errands, and temporarily stop speaking to our friends when they irritate us. Frankly, even the best relationships can be strained at times. You don't have to be fighting with your loved ones in order for them to stress you out, either. Perhaps you feel that you're having difficulty communicating with your girlfriend, or that there's some sort of fundamental difference of opinion that keeps you from being closer with your childhood best friend.

It can be hard to put aside personal grievances and conflicts, but Yoga can give you new peace and perspective. Generally, meditation helps you become more centered, thoughtful, and in touch with yourself. It enhances your perception of the world and your place in it. As a result, you're better equipped to connect with other people--more emotionally responsive and flexible, not only right after your session, but over the course of your day and week. When you yourself are in a better frame of mind, you'll find you're better able to accept others and be more tolerant of their foibles.

The specific meditations that follow will help you expand your ability to bear uncomfortable emotions by training your mind to stay focused on more positive feelings. As you focus your mind, you will be able to rise above petty disagreements and feel greater empathy and compassion for the people you care about. You'll find that you have an easier time putting yourself in your loved ones' shoes and understanding why they feel the way they do. Perhaps most important, you'll remember why you love your friends and family in the first place.

If you practice these meditations on a regular basis, with time, you'll find your stress levels decrease. You may even realize that you get angry or upset less frequently. And by cultivating a way of life in which you interact more sensitively with the people in your life who matter to you, you'll also be contributing to the greater harmony of your sangha, or community (see page 143).

42. Loving Kindness Meditation
Metta

BENEFITS

In the Dhammapada, a collection of sayings from the Buddha, there is a saying:

Never here by enmity
are those with enmity allayed,
they are allayed by amity,
this is the timeless truth.

The following meditation, called *metta,* is sort of the Buddhist version of turning the other cheek—a way of meeting hostility and anger with love and compassion. This deep meditation reconditions your mind, overriding your old, negative default patterns and installing new, positive ones. It also helps you feel more connected to others, more positive about your loved ones, and more accepting of yourself. The loving kindness meditation is so straightforward that children can easily perform it, but so profound that adults will find significant benefits.

TECHNIQUE

Sit comfortably and close your eyes. Begin by silently imagining what you wish for your own life. For instance, you may say to yourself, "May I be happy, may I be healthy and strong, may I be peaceful and joyful." Then move on to wishing the same things for someone you love. Next, affirm these good wishes for someone toward whom you have neutral feelings—a person you neither love nor hate. Then send these wishes to someone with whom you're having a hard time. Finally, send this loving kindness toward the whole universe and beyond!

DURATION

Do a fifteen-minute meditation every day for best results.

43. Rainbow Arc of Love

BENEFITS

The rainbow arc of love meditation is one of my favorites. It's actually a visualization in which you will be using your vivid imagination to see a rainbow in your mind's eye—and to send love through that rainbow to a person you love, or to a person with whom you've been experiencing emotional turmoil.

This meditation is so soothing that it's almost impossible to stay mad at someone after you practice it. I use this meditation to calm myself after a disagreement with a family member, friend, or coworker. The rainbow arc of love helps to dissipate the negative energy and the unkind, judgmental thoughts we're prone to when we think we're not being heard or not getting our way. It's also a sweet way to send loving energy to anyone you think might need it, even if you're not mad. My niece uses it to send energy to her son when he comes up to bat in Little League!

TECHNIQUE

Sit comfortably and close your eyes. Take a few deep calming breaths to center yourself. If you're really upset it may take more than a few breaths, so take more if you need them. Mentally check your face for tension. If you're frowning or furrowing your brow, allow your facial muscles to relax. Notice how your eyes feel—see if you can relax and soften them.

Mentally observe the rest of your body, and if you notice tension, let go and relax. Bring your awareness to your heart center, in your chest area. Then imagine the heart center of the person with whom you are connecting. See a rainbow of colors forming an arc from your heart to his or hers. Imagine this arc is radiant with love and light, compassion and tenderness. Keep in mind that these gentle qualities are coming from the highest source—from God if you will—rather than from you personally.

DURATION

A short session of ten to fifteen minutes can accomplish great healing, but you can continue at your own pace for as long as is comfortable. If you find the rainbow image fading away after a few moments, don't bother with it. Simply continue to sit quietly, concentrating on the feeling of love and acceptance.

ADAPTATION

If you're having trouble visualizing the rainbow, don't worry. Instead, it may be easier to start from darkness. With every inhalation, imagine that you are bringing more light into the darkness. With every exhalation, know that you are expelling the darkness from your mind and sending it back to the nothingness from whence it came. Once you feel the darkness has dissipated, continue with the rainbow arc of love.

Meditations for Illness or Injury

Illness and injury happen to all of us. When you get sick or hurt, it can feel as if your life has come to a halt. Whether the ailment is temporary or chronic, the effects can be devastating, making it difficult to function. It's even worse when you still have to fulfill all your responsibilities while you're not at your best. The pressure can be enormous. I know I find it challenging to be a good example of Yoga when I'm injured or not feeling one hundred percent. All of my work skills—singing, playing the piano, and teaching Yoga—require my body to be in good working order!

"Tomorrow's worry will make you sick today. Stay healthy today!"
—SWAMI SATCHIDANANDA

Fortunately, as I mentioned earlier, current studies show that meditation has powerful benefits, not only for your mind, but for your body, as well. With each passing year, new research confirms the healing powers of meditation. Scientists now believe that regular meditation somehow serves to boost the immune system, helping you fight off disease. One recent study conducted by Harvard Medical School researchers has suggested that mind-body techniques like meditation can actually switch on and off certain genes that regulate stress and the immune response.

But how can meditation help when you're already sick or in pain? Research suggests that in addition to alleviating depression and anxiety, meditation can help provide relief from a wide variety of physical ailments, including asthma, cancer, heart disease, irritable bowel syndrome, ulcerative colitis, chronic pain, and insomnia. Some studies have indicated that meditation may even lower blood pressure and reduce the likelihood, length, and severity of acute respiratory illnesses like the flu.

Clearly, meditation can help keep you healthy in more ways than one. In this section, I'll introduce you to a number of meditations that can make you feel better and allow you to take care of your obligations. These meditations focus on physical wellness, giving you a greater awareness of your body. With this greater awareness, you'll be able to target the sources of your discomfort and release any tensions or pains. Moreover, if you do these meditations consistently, you may be able to bolster your health and protect yourself from future illnesses or injuries.

44. Healing Affirmation

Pratipaksha Bhavana

BENEFITS

As you learned earlier, the first two branches of Patanjali's eight-limbed tree—yama and niyama—form a set of ten rules or "commandments" that every Yogi should follow. Some of these guidelines can be very useful to those of us who are struggling with illness or injury. One of the rules is to practice *santosha,* or contentment. In santosha, you are asked to accept life on life's terms, without resistance. To use the words of the Beatles, you simply "let it be." Another commandment is *tapas,* or austerity; in this context, tapas means that you should view any pain as a challenge that allows you to purify your mind and strengthen your will. Accept the pain as an act of surrender, or *ishvara pranidhana,* and understand that what happens to your body is in the hands of a higher power. We may not understand why accidents or illnesses happen, but we can have faith that the peace and joy that is our true self is everlasting, and that whatever pain we experience is transitory.

TECHNIQUE

Sitting comfortably, take a few deep breaths and tune in to your body. Observe your unpleasant symptoms and let them go. You are going to practice a technique called *pratipaksha bhavana.* In pratipaksha bhavana, you replace negative thoughts with positive thoughts. Whenever a negative thought comes up— "My arm is killing me," for example—turn it into a positive affirmation appropriate for the injury or ailment: "I see my arm completely healthy and strong," "My arm is filled with healing energy," or "Every breath I take is revitalizing my arm." Your positive message can be something more general, too: "I trust my body to heal." You can repeat your positive affirmation several times to allow its message sink deep into your consciousness. Or, if you have good powers of visualization, simply envision the healing happening, and hold that image in your mind's eye for a few minutes.

The "Ten Commandments" of Yoga

The first two limbs of the eight-limbed tree of Yoga (see page 113), *yama* and *niyama,* set forth basic rules of conduct that are intended to help keep the mind and body clean and calm. By following these rules, or "commandments," you aim to achieve—or at least approximate—ethical perfection and control of the mind and senses.

Yama

Yama, the Sanskrit word for restraint, informs five rules for dealing with the outside world, including:

1. *Ahimsa.* Nonviolence, respect for all life.

2. *Satya.* Truthfulness in word and deed.

3. *Asteya.* Nonstealing.

4. *Brahmacharya.* Continence or abstinence, moderation in all things.

5. *Aparigraha.* Avoidance of greed and coveting.

Niyama

Niyama, or "observance," informs five rules that apply to your personal life and behavior:

1. *Shaucha.* Purity.

2. *Santosha.* Contentment.

3. *Tapas.* Austerity and acceptance of pain.

4. *Svadhyaya.* Spiritual study and self-examination.

5. *Ishvara pranidhana.* Surrender to the Divine.

As you follow these ten commandments consistently, you'll become a shining example of Yoga! Everyone will want to know you and be around you, as you exude a charismatic joy and calmness.

DURATION

After you make your positive affirmation or visualization, sit with it for five to ten minutes. Then observe the peaceful feeling created by your practice, and allow your mind to rest. If your mind begins to wander or get fidgety, you can always bring it back to the affirmation or visualization.

If you find this meditation is helpful, sit with it a little longer, or for up to half an hour.

45. The Yogic Sleep

Yoga Nidra

BENEFIT

Also known as Yoga Nidra, Yogic sleep is a guided form of meditation that uses progressive relaxation to encourage better awareness of the mind and body. According to Yogic philosophy, the body is made of up five *koshas*—subtle coverings, or sheaths. There is the physical sheath, *annamaya kosha;* the energy sheath, *pranamaya kosha;* the sheath of the mind and senses, the *manomaya kosha;* the sheath of higher wisdom, the *vijnanamaya kosha;* and the bliss sheath, the *anandamaya kosha.* Yoga Nidra allows us to rest and heal these more elusive parts of ourselves as we systematically relax each sheath or body from the outside in.

Yoga Nidra reduces stress in the muscles and organs, and helps stabilize the parasympathetic nervous system—the part of the nervous system that controls certain automatic bodily functions, including arousal, digestion, heart rate, and defecation. This form of meditation can be especially effective in helping the body right itself and facilitate healing on the physical level, the annamaya kosha. It can also alleviate mental strain and help to heal old emotional scars that may be held in the manomaya kosha.

TECHNIQUE

It's best to do this meditation on a moderately empty stomach. Go somewhere where you will not be disturbed for the next twenty minutes. Close the door and turn off your phone. Put on an extra sweater or drape a blanket around your shoulders, as your body temperature will drop during the meditation and you don't want to get a chill. If possible, lie on your back with your legs and arms spread out to your sides, palms facing up. This is the supine corpse pose, or *savasana.* Feel that the floor is doing all the work of supporting your body—you're not holding on anywhere. Rest deeply, but try not to fall asleep.

Let's begin. Focus your attention on your right leg—stretch it out, lift it a couple inches from the floor, and point your toes. Squeeze your right leg tight and then suddenly relax, letting your leg drop as if it were a branch cut from a tree. Roll your leg gently from side to side—and then forget about it. Repeat with your left leg:

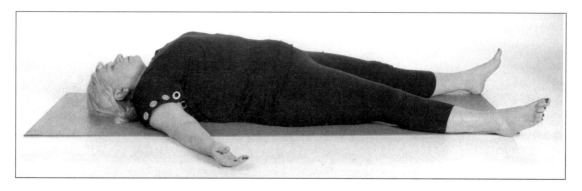

stretch it out, lift it off the floor, point your toes, and tense all the muscles in your leg, and then release them.

Continue in the same manner with your right arm. Stretch out the fingers on your right hand and tighten your whole arm, lifting it a few inches off the ground. Make a fist and squeeze it tight. Make your arm longer and tighter, and then relax, dropping your arm to the ground. Roll your right arm gently from side to side, and then forget about it. Shift your attention to your left arm, and repeat the process.

Move on to your buttocks: squeeze them tight, almost as if you're about to rise right up off the floor. Then release the tension. Shift your focus to your belly. Inhale deeply, as if you were filling a big balloon. Take in as much air as you can hold, letting your belly stick all the way out. Hold your breath in your belly for a moment, then open your mouth and let the air gush out. Inhale again, this time into your upper chest; hold briefly, then open your mouth and exhale.

Now observe your shoulders. Shrug them up toward your ears, squeeze them tight, then release. Next, bring your shoulders forward, as if to make them touch under your chin. Squeeze, then let your shoulders drop. Now move on to your face. Open your mouth, stick out your tongue, stretch out all the muscles of your face, and then release. Now make a prune face, tightening all your facial muscles, and then release. Gently roll your head from side to side once or twice, releasing any tension in your neck. Then bring your head back to its normal, central position.

Take a moment to observe your body, and make any minor adjustments to your savasana pose. You might need to scratch your nose, wiggle the shoulders, or widen the stance of your legs for greater comfort. Mentally check your body and make sure that you aren't holding tension anywhere. You are going to go over your body again, this time without moving a single muscle, so if you feel you need to make an adjustment, do it now. You don't want to keep adjusting throughout the next bit of the process.

You'll be deepening your relaxation mentally, beginning at your feet. Check the bottoms of your feet for any residual tension, and let it melt away. Check your toes. If there is any tension there, gently release it. Continue in this way, relaxing the tops of your feet, your arches, heels, and ankles. Then move into your legs, relaxing your shins, calves, knees, backs of your knees, and thighs. Move your awareness to your hands, forearms, and upper arms. If you find any rebellious muscle that is holding on, let it go. Relax your buttocks, hips, and groin. Relax your belly, rib cage, upper chest, and all your internal organs. Observe the back of your body and relax your spine, shoulder blades, shoulders, and neck. Relax all the parts of your head, from the jaw up to the crown of your head. Relax your lips, tongue, nose, and eyes. Relax your eyebrows and the space between your eyebrows. Relax your ears and temples. Relax.

Take a moment to observe the peaceful feeling in your body. Make note of it so you can refer to this feeling any time you start to notice yourself tensing up. Then observe your breath for a minute or two. Your breath will have become very quiet, almost imperceptible. Don't try to change or control it, just watch. Pause here as you observe your breath. Then move your attention to your mind. Notice how your mind feels very still and quiet, too. Whenever thoughts arise, just let them float away; don't get too interested in them. Become a witness to your mind. By doing this, you access your true self— your essential consciousness or awareness, which is above judgments and evaluations and beyond pairs of opposites like good and bad, profit and loss, rich and poor. Rest easy. Stay in this restful state for another five or ten minutes before waking your body. Try not to fall asleep.

To wake your body, begin by bringing your mind back. Gradually deepen your breaths, and your body will naturally want to wake up. Take all the time you need. Gently bring your body back to an active state, wiggling your fingers and toes, and having a nice stretch, as if you've just had a power nap.

When you feel ready, roll over to one side, pause here for a moment or two, and at your own pace, gradually come back to a seated position. Keep your eyes closed

"The investigation that occurs during Yoga Nidra inevitably leads to the deconstruction and disidentification of our basic core beliefs about who we take ourselves to be. As our beliefs and assumptions dissolve, we glimpse our essential Nature as Presence and come to the firsthand conviction that we are not the limited, finite creatures that we mistakenly take ourselves to be. We find, instead, that we are a Vastness unfathomable to the mind; a joyous Beingness that is always present, even in the midst of the greatest difficulty. This is the supreme understanding that Yoga Nidra invites us to realize."

—RICHARD MILLER, CLINICAL PSYCHOLOGIST
AND YOGA SCHOLAR

for another minute or two, observing the peaceful feeling created by your Yoga Nidra practice. If you have time, you can do some pranayama before going back into your day. This tranquil experience of the true self is available to you at any time, in any place, because the true self is you! It may be hard to imagine getting to that state of awareness, but eventually you will be able to experience a joy and peace of mind you may never have known before.

DURATION

Try to allow at least twenty to thirty minutes for this rejuvenating practice.

ADAPTATION

If you're not comfortable lying on the floor in a supine position, you can do this entire sequence seated on a chair. Scoot your buttocks to the back of the chair so that your spine is perpendicular to the seat of the chair; place your feet on the floor and your hands on your thighs. Now you're ready to begin.

Note: Instead of memorizing all the steps, many people find it useful to listen to a recording of instructions for Yoga Nidra. You can download a free audio guide to this practice at www.BigYogaForLessStress.com.

Meditations for Money Problems

Money is a major source of anxiety for many people. Maybe you're working at a job that is paying the bills but robbing you of your vitality. Maybe you've lost a job or become homeless. Maybe you've recently retired and are wondering if you can live comfortably on a fixed income. Or maybe you've become overburdened with debt and can't find a way out. In this day and age, more and more people are facing economic insecurity, finding it difficult to cover expenses and provide for their families—never mind setting a little money aside in savings. Because money is such a critical component of everyday life, it can be hard to remember that it isn't everything, and that you have a spiritual and emotional existence that extends beyond your capacity as an income-earner.

In this section, I will show you a meditation and a few other Yogic strategies that may be able to help you. While these strategies won't magically deliver thousands of dollars into your bank account, they may provide some relief from your financial stress. As I explained earlier, meditation allows you to cultivate a greater sense of perspective. Once you realize that many obstacles are temporary and can be overcome, your troubles will seem more manageable.

It's important to be kind to yourself, no matter what your circumstances are. God—the cosmic consciousness, the creator, or whatever name you'd like to give to the higher power—has a plan for you. Not that you have to believe in God to benefit from the exercises I show you here. Studies have shown that even those who don't believe in God find that their outlook on life is improved by the perception that their lives have purpose. And your life does have purpose. You are so much more than the money you make. Remember that each of us has a place in the universe, and take comfort in that thought.

46. Meditation for Prosperity

BENEFITS

We all have what's known in Sanskrit as *samskaras*—grooves in our minds where thoughts naturally fall. When you're worried, these grooves can perpetuate negativity. For example, if you're going through hard times, you may have a repeating thought of "I can't afford to pay my bills." In this meditation, you will cultivate a steadier, more positive outlook on your finances by installing new, healthier grooves in place of the old, negative grooves.

TECHNIQUE

Sitting comfortably, close your eyes and take a few deep breaths. Steer your thoughts to the space around your heart. Silently tell yourself, "My life is blessed with abundance," and envision your heart glowing with a soft golden light. Now expand that light outward, imagining that the golden light is infusing every cell in your body. Silently tell yourself, "All obstacles to receiving wealth are being removed by the light."

Next, observe the area around your body and affirm to yourself, "All thought of lack is being dissolved into the light." Keep expanding that light outwards. Say, "I bring prosperity into my life."

Imagine the light extending further and shining brighter, until the room you are in is enveloped in golden light. Stay in this sacred, lighted space for as long as you like. Then, begin to bring the light back in to your heart center. Imagine that the light is being reabsorbed into your heart. To return to normal consciousness, bless your surroundings by affirming, "May the entire universe be blessed with happiness, prosperity, and health." Notice the comforting effect of your meditation.

DURATION

Take as much time as you need to create your glowing sphere of light, and take as much time as you need to bring the light back to your heart center As you maintain your focus on your heart center, enjoy the peaceful feeling you've created.

47. Laughter Yoga

Hasyayoga

BENEFITS

Swami Satchidananda often said that laughter is the best medicine. He used humor in his talks to keep us from taking ourselves too seriously—as young Yoga students, we were trying so hard to become "enlightened" that sometimes we just needed a little fun!

Technically, laughter Yoga is more a method of relaxation than it is a formal meditation. But it is a very useful technique that can provide much-needed stress relief and help bring perspective to your troubles, whether they are financial or social in nature. The benefits of laughter have been scientifically demonstrated. Laughing helps to release endorphins—special feel-good chemicals—in your brain. These endorphins work to improve your mood and reduce stress on both an emotional and physical level. Moreover, laughter Yoga strengthens the immune system and brings more oxygen to the body and brain. It is therapeutic, but it also helps prevent future recurrences of stress and even disease. Finally, you can see laughter Yoga almost as a form of exercise, giving the heart a cardiovascular workout and massage. Regular laughter Yoga can help dilate your blood vessels, allowing blood to flow more freely.

TECHNIQUE

Laughter Yoga amounts to laughing for no reason. If you can't find anything funny to get you going, start with fake laughter and keep laughing until you laugh for real! Your body can't tell if you're laughing out of genuine amusement or faking it—you still get the benefits. It's good to do this type of "meditation" with a group. Trying to sustain a laughing session for fifteen minutes is difficult to do on your own! Besides, laughter is contagious, and there are advantages to spending time with others socially—in *sangha,* the Sanskrit word for community of believers— that enhance the basic benefits of laughter. You can find laughter Yoga classes at colleges, Yoga studios, and dedicated laughter clubs. If you have recently retired, look for a laughter Yoga class at your local senior center.

At a laughter Yoga session, the leader will gather everyone in a circle. You'll be encouraged to make eye contact, which is important in stimulating "fake" laughter.

The leader might begin with some laughter exercises and a few jokes to get the group warmed up. Soon you will feel less inhibited and start laughing for no reason. After about fifteen minutes of these laughter exercises, the leader might have everyone lie head to head on the floor, bodies stretching out like the spokes of a large wheel. You will be encouraged to keep laughing at your own pace. Don't worry—you'll find it easy to keep going when you hear the wide variety of guffaws, giggles, hoots, hollers, and shrieks that fill the room! The session usually closes with a guided progressive relaxation. When the whole session is over, you will be completely rejuvenated!

DURATION

I recommend laughing by yourself for fifteen to thirty minutes, two or three times each week. Alternatively, you can simply attend a group session once a week.

48. Chanting and Kirtan

BENEFITS

Like laughter, singing and chanting are uplifting practices that stimulate your heart and improve your mood. The deep breathing required for singing also brings more prana into your system, and the long, extended exhalations help retain the prana. In addition, when you sing in a group, your body releases oxytocin—the "cuddle" hormone—a chemical that enhances feelings of trust and bonding and lowers anxiety and stress.

TECHNIQUE

If you're going solo, pick a song or chant that inspires you. It can be devotional, plaintive, or celebratory, according to your mood. As we discussed in our section on mantras, one of the simplest and most profound chants is om shanti. According to Yogic teaching, "om" is the sound of the universe, a sound from which all other sounds (and matter) are formed, a cosmic hum that connects you to your source. "Shanti" is the Sanskrit word meaning peace, but it also evokes peace when you chant it out loud or even repeat it mentally. Saying this phrase over and over is guaranteed to create a serene feeling. In general, chanting is begun at a moderate tempo, and continues with slight variations in speed, according to your mood. You can pick any pitch that feels comfortable to you as your starting point. It's fine to vary your pitch from time to time, too. If

> "If you chant the names of God with a loving and open heart, all the secrets of the name come out to you. Like a shower or a waterfall, it pours its grace into you."
> —KARNAMRITA DAS

you are using the om shanti chant, feel free to try the three different melodies I've provided. Once you begin the chant, proceed without any breaks or pauses until you're ready to stop. When you chant, imagine blessings of peace flowing into you and going out into the world. You can listen to an example of this chant at www.BigYogaForLessStress.com.

Looking for inspiration or further instruction? You can listen to or chant along with CDs or audio files of various contemporary chant artists. For some recommendations, check the Resources section in the back of the book. Or, if you'd like to familiarize yourself with chanting or join a group, go to your local Yoga studio when

Om Shanti

Here is a simple tune that we use at the ashram to chant om shanti. It has three basic melodies; one high, one low, and one in the middle:

Start out slowly, bringing your awareness to the sound of the mantra. As your voice warms up, gradually speed up the tempo. Chant a little louder! Try improvising on the basic melody—it's okay to be creative. Con-tinue for as long as you like. When you're ready, begin to slow the tempo down and chant a little softer, until you're feeling the peaceful vibration of the shanti mantra. Fin-ish the chant and sit quietly, repeating the mantra silently. End your session with a short affirmation—for example, "The ben-efits of my chanting will bring peace and har-mony to all."

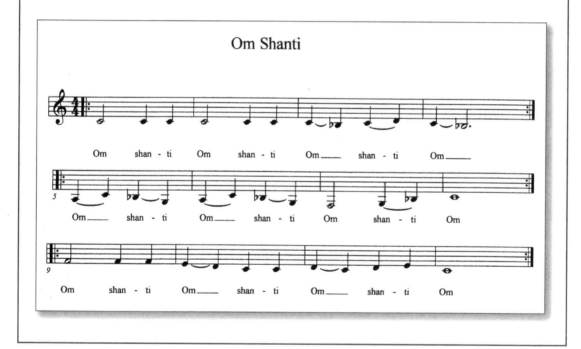

Om Shanti

they're hosting an evening of *kirtan* to experience the profound sense of joy and sweetness that is elicited by chanting together. Kirtan is a special form of organized chanting that is usually done in a call and response manner, following a leader, or *kirtan wallah*. If you prefer western music, find a church, synagogue, or community choir that you can join. You will enjoy both the feeling of community (sangha) and the element of devotion.

If you prefer to use a more traditional approach, try singing a simple song you learned in childhood, such as "He's Got the Whole World in His Hands" or the Shaker hymn "Simple Gifts." You can use any uplifting song—it can be devotional, plaintive, or celebratory, according to your mood.

As I explained earlier, you can sing by yourself, or you can sing in a group. You can also sing a cappella (without accompaniment) or you can sing along with a drum, tambourine, guitar, or keyboard.

DURATION

If you're alone, try chanting for up to fifteen minutes. With a group, a half-hour or hour-long session is terrific.

The Importance of Community

One important element in Yoga is the idea of *sangha,* or the community of the faithful. Spending time with people who love and support you in your Yoga quest can be immensely helpful if you are stressed out or going through hard times. Keep up with your friends, or perhaps make some new ones! An excellent way to do this is by performing good works within your community. The discipline of Karma Yoga, the so-called "Yoga of action," teaches us to provide selfless service to the world as a way of rising above our stress. In Karma Yoga, you offer the fruits of your labor to the higher good, allowing your ego—both the shaming ego and the boastful ego— to go on vacation. You feel that you are an instrument in the hands of the Divine. Community service gives those of us who are stressed some much-needed perspective, reminding us that there is a world outside our personal problems.

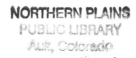

Conclusion

I hope that this book has inspired you to make Yoga a part of your daily routine. Yoga is not about shutting yourself up in a cave or at an ashram—you don't have to give up pleasure. As you learned earlier, Yoga is about making good choices and improving your well-being. The idea is to get into a regular habit of doing Yoga poses, breathing practices, and meditation. In this way, Yoga can become a stabilizing force in your constantly changing life.

Yoga empowers you to manage the negative impact of stress. Stress affects us on so many levels, hurting us physically, mentally, emotionally, and even spiritually. Taking on just one simple Yoga practice—such as ten minutes of pranayama each day—can help. It's as if you're pulling on a string that's connected to the different levels of stress, releasing all your anxiety, unhappiness, and exhaustion. Any tension you might have had will begin to melt away, and you will be able to meet difficult situations head on, with full confidence. With your newly focused, meditative mind, you'll find that solutions to hard problems will present themselves effortlessly. And nothing is ever lost. If you have to take a break from your practice for a while, don't worry. When you're able to get back to your Yoga routine, it will feel like an old friend.

The techniques I've shown you in this book can also strengthen your will, allowing you, in the words of Buddhist author Pema Chödrön, to "investigate the strategies of the ego." The ego uses many tricky methods to pull you out of the present moment and make you worry about the future or ruminate about the past. In a way, that's the ego's job—to judge and evaluate your experiences—but it's easy to let your mind slip into a repetitive, negative groove that isn't helpful. With the resilience that comes with ongoing Yoga practice, you can coax the mind and ego back into the present moment, where all the fun is! It is in the golden present that you tune in to something profound within yourself. Through the ancient practices of Yoga, you can bring yourself back into the peace and serenity that is your true nature.

According to the Yogis, each of us is made of pure spirit, and this spirit is part of the infinite consciousness. When we discover we are one with the universe, we realize that there is nothing that separates us from anyone and anything, and so there is no reason for fighting or discord. Yoga teaches us to rise above our judgments and foster equanimity, encouraging us to treat others—and ourselves—with compassion and love. With this in mind, as my guru used to say, we can create a heaven on earth.

Let's do that. Let's keep ourselves calm. Let's radiate peace and love so that we can bring sweetness and joy to our families, our workplaces, and our world. With all the challenges facing our planet today, there has never been a better time to become a beacon of peace. My guru Swami Satchidananda felt that each one of us should affirm to ourselves, "Peace on earth begins with me." Won't you take up the challenge? Begin practicing Yoga today—the world needs you!

Glossary

ahimsa. Nonviolence; one of the five yamas.

anjali mudra. Common mudra used in prayer and in greeting, hands pressed together at the heart center.

aparigraha. Avoidance of greed and coveting; one of the five yamas.

asana. A comfortable, steady posture that promotes a feeling of stillness within.

ashram. A Hindu term for a religious retreat where students are guided by spiritually qualified, ordained swamis.

Ashtanga Yoga. The eight-fold path of Yoga as described in Patanjali's Yoga Sutras, including yama, niyama, asana, pranayama, pratyhara, dharana, dhyana, and samadhi.

asteya. Nonstealing; one of the five yamas.

Bhakti Yoga. The Yoga of devotion and love.

brahmacharya. Continence or abstinence; moderation in all things; one of the five yamas.

Brahman. The universal self.

dandasana. Staff pose; a sitting position in which your legs are extended out in front and your hands are placed slightly behind your body, supporting it.

dharma. The path of righteousness; your spiritual duty.

guru. Remover of darkness; one who is spiritually enlightened and able to help devotees uncover their own inner lights.

Hatha. A form of Yoga that emphasizes the creation of balance. The term is often used to denote the use of asanas alone, but Hatha Yoga includes many other practices, including pranayama.

ishvara pranidhana. Surrender to the divine; one of the five niyamas.

japa. Continuous chanting or recitation of a mantra or prayer.

Karma Yoga. The Yoga of action; emphasizes need to provide selfless service to the world.

kirtan. The practice of chanting the names of God.

kirtan wallah. Chant leader.

koshas. The coverings or sheaths of the physical and astral bodies.

kriya. Cleansing practice.

mahasamadhi. The soul's conscious exit from the body.

mala beads. Special prayer necklaces that can aid concentration and meditation.

mandala. Sacred geometric symbol.

mantra. Sound structure that settles the mind; incantation.

moksha. Pure, undifferentiated consciousness, a state of bliss.

mudra. Seal; gesture used to seal energy in the body.

nadi. Subtle energy channel found throughout the body, similar to a meridian in acupuncture.

niyama. The second limb of Patanjali's eight-limbed Yoga tree. It encompasses five Yogic observances or disciplines, including purity, contentment, austerity, study, and devotion.

om. The name of the sound of the subtle vibration of the universe, from which all matter is created; the chief mantra.

prana. Vital energy, life force.

pranayama. Breathing techniques used to control (yama) vital energy (prana).

pratyahara. The fifth limb on Patanjali's Yoga tree; the discipline of withdrawing the mind from the senses.

Raja Yoga. The royal path of Yoga, as outlined in Patanjali's Yoga Sutras; practices leading to mastery of the mind and senses.

rishi. Ancient seer.

samadhi. The most advanced state in Yoga, in which concentration merges with the object of concentration; a complete absorption in God or supreme consciousness.

samskara. Mental groove; impression that comes to your consciousness from your senses. It helps form the basis for your habits and beliefs.

sangha. Community of the faithful.

sankalpa. Firm decision; vow.

Sanskrit. Ancient liturgical language used in many important texts describing Yoga.

santosha. Contentment; one of the five niyamas.

satya. Truthfulness; one of the five yamas.

savasana. Corpse pose; a pose in which you lie supine, on your back.

shanti. The peace of God "that passes all understanding."

shaucha. Purity; one of the five niyamas.

so-hum. The mantra of the breath, so (the inhale) hum (the exhale) is roughly translated to mean "I am He."

sukhasana. Easy cross-legged position for meditation.

sutra. Literally, "thread." The Yoga Sutras are nearly 200 aphorisms compiled by the sage and physician Patanjali in the second or third century AD.

svadhyaya. Spiritual study and self-examination; one of the five niyamas.

swami. A monk, renunciate, or spiritual master.

tadasana. Mountain pose; a standing position in which your feet are about a foot apart and your arms are at your sides, palms facing inward.

tapas. Austerity; one of the five rules of niyama.

ujjayi. The hissing breath, caused by gently closing the glottis.

utkatasana. Chair pose; a standing position in which you hover as if about to sit on a chair.

vajrasana. Thunderbolt pose; a sitting position in which you sit with your heels tucked under you and your shins and the tops of your feet pressed against the floor.

Vedanta. A school of philosophy based on Vedic scripture, which believes in the Oneness of All; nondualism.

Vedas. Four ancient texts (Rig, Yajur, Sama, and Atharva) revealed to ancient sages and saints of India, and which explain every aspect of human life and the life divine.

vinyasa. Series of postures in a flow.

Vishnu mudra. Sacred mudra associated with Vishnu, the Hindu preserver of the universe.

yantra. A mystical diagram.

yama. The first limb Patanjali's Yoga tree. It encompasses a set of five Yogic abstinences, including nonviolence, truthfulness, non-stealing, chastity, and non-greed.

Yoga. From the Sanskrit words meaning to yoke or join together; uniting body, mind, and spirit.

Yoga Nidra. Restorative deep relaxation in which the body and mind are at rest, but not asleep in the normal sense.

zafu. Special meditation pillow.

Resources

In this book, I have shared various Yoga practices that have been shown to reduce or eliminate stress. I've included this Resources section in case you would like to explore any of the subjects I've discussed in greater detail. Here, you'll find my recommendations for books, instructional DVDs, CDs, ashrams, and websites.

RECOMMENDED READING

There's always more to learn about the ancient and evolving traditions of Yoga. In this section, I share with you some of my favorite books on meditation, relaxation, and Yoga technique. I hope they inspire you as much as they've inspired me!

Autobiography of a Yogi by Paramahansa Yogananda.

Beyond Words by Sri Swami Satchidananda.

Big Yoga: A Simple Guide for Bigger Bodies by Meera Patricia Kerr.

Breath By Breath by Larry Rosenberg.

Full Catastrophe Living: Using the Wisdom of Your Body and Mind to Face Stress, Pain, and Illness by Jon Kabat-Zinn.

The Genie in Your Genes by Dawson Church.

The Healing Path of Yoga by Nischala Joy Devi.

How God Changes Your Brain by Andrew Newberg and Mark Waldman.

Integral Yoga Hatha by Sri Swami Satchidananda.

The Joy of Yoga, edited by Jennifer Schwamm Willis.

Light on Pranayama by B.K.S. Iyengar.

Meditation and Its Practice by Swami Rama.

The Miracle of Mindfulness: A Manual on Meditation by Thich Nhat Hanh.

Present Moment, Wonderful Moment by Thich Nhat Hanh.

Relax and Renew: Restful Yoga for Stressful Times by Judith Lasater.

The Relaxation Response by Herbert Benson.

The Spectrum by Dean Ornish.

The Stress of Life by Hans Selye.

The Tapping Solution by Nick Ortner.

Yoga and the Quest for the True Self by Stephen Cope.

Yoga Nidra by Swami Satyananda Saraswati.

The Yoga Sutras of Patanjali by Sri Swami Satchidananda.

DVDS FOR HOME PRACTICE

For many of us, it's easier to learn by watching than by reading a book. These days, anybody can go to YouTube and watch a recorded Yoga class from any of a number of traditions. There are also sites that offer free streaming Yoga sessions. But for those of you who are still kicking it old school, here are a handful of instructional DVDs that you might find helpful as you get started in your practice. Included in my selection are DVDs that address the challenges faced by those of us with bigger bodies.

Accessible Yoga for Every Body by Susan Ward.

Bed Top Yoga by Carol Dickman.

Big Yoga: Flex-Ability by Meera Patricia Kerr.

Big Yoga: Hatha One by Meera Patricia Kerr.

Deepening Your Meditation by Swami Satchidananda.

Insight Yoga by Sarah Powers.

Integral Yoga: Yoga for Active Mature Populations by Manjula Spears.

Laugh-a-Yoga by Bharata Wingham.

CDS FOR GUIDED PRACTICE

The CDs listed below will guide you through your meditations. You may feel relaxed just listening to the soothing voices and quiet music!

Breathe to Beat the Blues by Amy Weintraub.

Deep Relaxation: Stress Management and Healing by Nischala Joy Devi.

Dynamic Stillness: Meditation Guidance by Nischala Joy Devi.

Guided Meditation by Swami Satchidananda.

How to Meditate by Pema Chödrön.

Meditation for Beginners by Jack Kornfield.

The Yoga of Sleep by Rubin Naiman.

KIRTAN AND CHANTING CDS

Want to hear how beautiful chanting can be? Here are a few CDs featuring some of my favorite kirtan wallahs (chant leaders). This is just a sampling of their work! If you like what you hear, you might want to check out a bhakti festival—a celebration of Yogic devotional singing. There may be one near you!

Best of Both Worlds by Ragani.

Bhakti Fest by various artists.

Embrace by Deva Premal.

Integral Yoga Kirtan by Swami Satchidananda.

Japa by Dave Stringer.

Kirtan! by Jai Uttal.

Live on Earth by Krishna Das.

Love Holding Love by Wah!

Sharanam by Sharon Gannon.

YOGA ASHRAMS

Once you start to practice Yoga regularly, you may find yourself wanting a deeper experience. A weekend retreat to an ashram (yoga center) may be just what you need to immerse yourself in the Yoga lifestyle.

Ananda Ashram
Yoga Society of New York
13 Sapphire Road
Monroe, NY 10950
www.anandaashram.org
(845) 782-5575

Amrit Yoga Institute
23855 NE County Road 314
Salt Springs, FL 32134
www.amrityoga.org
(352) 685-3001

Himalayan Institute
952 Bethany Turnpike
Honesdale, PA 18431
www.himalayaninstitute.org
(800) 822-4547
(570) 253-5551

Kripalu Center for Yoga and Health
PO Box 309
Stockbridge, MA 01262
www.kripalu.org
(866) 200-5203

Mount Madonna Center
445 Summit Road
Watsonville, CA 95076
www.mountmadonna.org
(408) 846-4064

Satchidananda Ashram at Yogaville
108 Yogaville Way
Buckingham, VA 23921
www.yogaville.org
(434) 969-2048

Sivananda Ashram Yoga Retreat
PO Box N7550
Paradise Island, Nassau, Bahamas
www.sivanandabahamas.org
(416) 479-0199

WEBSITES

Today, there are hundreds of reliable online resources for learning more about Yoga. Here are a few of my favorite websites.

www.BhaktiFest.com
Bhakti Fest's website primarily provides information on their Yoga, dance, and music festivals and retreats, but also offers educational information and videos.

www.CurvyYoga.com
Author and yoga teacher Anna Guest-Jelley reaches out to people of all sizes with her blog.

www.DianneBondyYoga.com
The website of educator Dianne Bondy provides webcasts and blog posts about Yoga with a special focus on diversity of size and color.

www.ElephantJournal.com
Elephant Journal is an online magazine that is dedicated to the "mindful life," providing articles and videos on Yoga, organic living, spirituality, and environmental awareness.

www.Heart.org
The American Heart Association's website has a whole subdivision devoted to stress management.

www.HuffingtonPost.com/ healthy-living
This section of the Huffington Post provides up-to-date articles about health and fitness, and often has content on the subjects of Yoga and stress management.

www.IYDbooks.com
Integral Yoga Distribution is a website that sells Yoga books, CDs, DVDs, and accessories. Many of their items are otherwise hard to get in the United States!

www.MindBodyGreen.com
MindBodyGreen is an online magazine that focuses on natural health and wellness.

www.OrnishSpectrum.com
The website of eminent doctor Dean Ornish offers lots of information on managing stress through approaches like Yoga and meditation.

www.ResilienceForLife.com
The site of stress management coach Jaymie Meyer has an extensive resources section where you can read inspiring articles and listen to audio files guiding you through various pranayama and deep relaxation techniques.

www.Stress.org
The American Institute of Stress's website contains many free recent articles, publications, podcasts, and videos about the effects of stress on daily life and health.

www.WholeLiving.com
Whole Living is a website that offers information on living a natural, sustainable lifestyle, and features many articles on Yoga and stress relief.

www.YogaAccessories.com
Yoga Accessories is a great resource for all your Yoga product needs. They offer high-quality mats, straps, locks, pillows, and other accessories at reasonable prices.

www.YogaDork.com
Yoga Dork provides current information on Yoga trends and practices. The site also reviews new Yoga books, videos, CDs, and movies.

www.YogaInternational.com
Yoga International offers articles and videos on Yoga. Online Yoga classes are also available for a small monthly membership fee.

www.YogaJournal.com
This site is the online edition of the magazine *Yoga Journal*. It provides free articles and video tutorials on Yoga poses and practices.

www.Yoganonymous.com
This site offers free online classes, music playlists, tips, and other information on Yoga practices and events.

Index

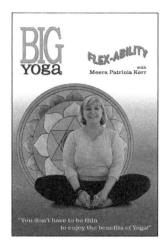
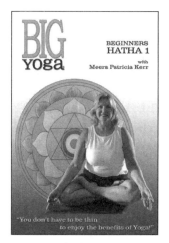
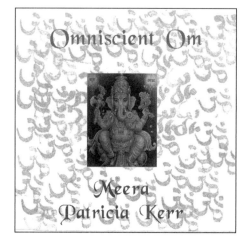

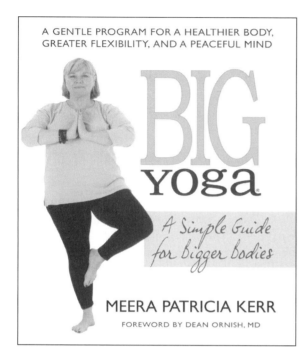

A GENTLE PROGRAM FOR A HEALTHIER BODY, GREATER FLEXIBILITY, AND A PEACEFUL MIND

$17.95
240 pages
7.5 x 9-inch quality paperback
ISBN 978-0-7570-0215-1

BIG YOGA
A Simple Guide for Bigger Bodies
Meera Patricia Kerr

If you think Yoga is only for skinny young things, you need to think again. To expert Meera Patricia Kerr, Yoga can be used by anyone—including those with bigger bodies. With an emphasis on health and relaxation, Meera has developed a unique Yoga program for larger individuals. In *Big Yoga*, she shares her successful plan with all those who think that Yoga is not for them.

Part One of *Big Yoga* begins with a clear explanation of what Yoga is, what benefits it offers, and how it can fit into anyone's life. Included is an important discussion of self-image. The book goes on to provide practical information regarding clothing, mats, and suitable environments, and to emphasize the need to begin your Yoga practice with care. Part Two offers over forty different postures specifically designed to work with bigger bodies. In each case, Meera explains the benefit of the posture and offers step-by-step instructions. Easy-to-follow photographs accompany every exercise, as well.

If you have thought that Yoga is not for you, pick up *Big Yoga* and let Meera Patricia Kerr help you become more confident, relaxed, and healthy than you may have ever thought possible.

THE DŌ-IN WAY
Gentle Exercises to Liberate the Body, Mind, and Spirit
Michio Kushi

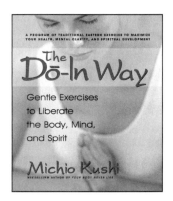

Dō-In is an ancient traditional exercise for the cultivation of physical health, mental serenity, and spirituality. Over the last 5,000 years, it has served as the origin of such well-known disciplines as shiatsu, acupuncture, moxibustion, yogic exercises, and meditation. Literally meaning to pull and stretch, Dō-In originated as a way of achieving longevity and attaining the highest potential of mental and spiritual development.

Dō-In techniques are a series of successive motions designed to harmonize body systems. *The Dō-In Way* details the fundamental aspects of this exercise, which involves breathing, posture, and self-massage and manipulation to stimulate body systems. The gentle application of pressure on the body's meridians corresponds directly with physical processes, and allows for the conditioning and stimulation of internal organs. This is a comprehensive handbook to an ancient system of movement designed to enhance physical, mental, and spiritual health.

$15.95 US • 224 pages • 7.5 x 9-inch quality paperback • ISBN 978-0-7570-0268-7

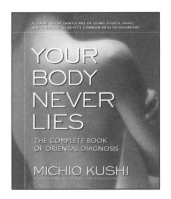

YOUR BODY NEVER LIES
The Complete Book of Oriental Diagnosis
Michio Kushi

Too often, conventional medicine fails to detect illness—especially when it first begins and is easiest to cure. But Oriental diagnosis, an ancient holistic system of knowledge, can often discover physical problems even before they arise. Now *Your Body Never Lies* helps you both understand and use this natural, noninvasive approach to restoring good health.

Your Body Never Lies starts by explaining the principles of Oriental medicine. It then shows you how to detect and understand health problems simply by looking at the mouth, lips, and teeth; eyes; nose, cheeks, and ears; forehead; hair; hands; feet; and skin. Clear diagrams and easy-to-use charts assist you in quickly recognizing signs of illness so that you can begin working toward a state of balanced well-being. Here is a complete guide to Oriental diagnosis, a revolutionary yet centuries-old way to identify and prevent disease while preserving health and harmony.

$16.95 • 184 pages • 7.5 x 9-inch quality paperback • ISBN 978-0-7570-0267-0

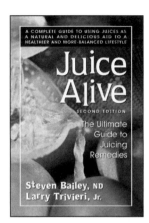

JUICE ALIVE, SECOND EDITION
The Ultimate Guide to Juicing Remedies
Steven Bailey, ND and Larry Trivieri, Jr.

The world of fresh juices offers a powerhouse of antioxidants, vitamins, minerals, and enzymes. The trick is knowing which juices can best serve your needs. In this easy-to-use guide, health experts Dr. Steven Bailey and Larry Trivieri, Jr. tell you everything you need to know to maximize the benefits and tastes of juice.

The book begins with a look at the history of juicing. It then examines the many components that make fresh juice truly good for you—good for weight loss and so much more. Next, it offers practical advice about the types of juices available, as well as buying and storing tips for produce. The second half of the book begins with an important chart that matches up common ailments with the most appropriate juices, followed by over 100 delicious juice recipes. Let *Juice Alive* introduce you to a world bursting with the incomparable tastes and benefits of fresh juice.

$14.95 • 288 pages • 6 x 9-inch quality paperback • ISBN 978-0-7570-0266-3

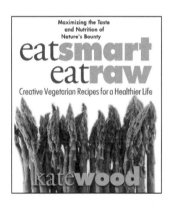

EAT SMART EAT RAW
Creative Vegetarian Recipes for a Healthier Life
Kate Wood

From healing diseases to detoxifying your body, from lowering cholesterol to eliminating excess weight, the many important health benefits derived from a raw vegetarian diet are too important to ignore. However, now there is another compelling reason to go raw—taste! In her new book *Eat Smart, Eat Raw,* cook and health writer Kate Wood not only explains how to get started, but also provides delicious kitchen-tested recipes guaranteed to surprise and delight even the fussiest of eaters.

Eat Smart, Eat Raw begins by explaining the basics of cooking without heat, from choosing the best equipment to stocking your pantry. What follows are twelve recipe chapters filled with truly exceptional dishes, including hearty breakfasts, savory soups, satisfying entrées, and luscious desserts.

$15.95 US • 184 pages • 7.5 x 9-inch quality paperback • ISBN 978-0-7570-0261-8

GOING WILD IN THE KITCHEN
The Fresh & Sassy Tastes of Vegetarian Cooking
Leslie Cerier

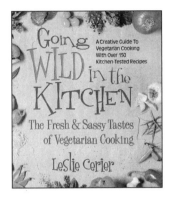

Going Wild in the Kitchen is the first comprehensive global vegetarian cookbook to go beyond the standard organic beans, grains, and vegetables. In addition to providing helpful cooking tips and techniques, the book contains over 150 kitchen-tested recipes for healthful, taste-tempting dishes—creative masterpieces that contain such unique ingredients as edible flowers; sea vegetables; and wild mushrooms, berries, and herbs. It encourages the creative side of novice and seasoned cooks alike, prompting them to follow their instincts and "go wild" in the kitchen by adding, changing, or substituting ingredients in existing recipes. To help, a wealth of suggestions is found throughout. A list of organic food sources completes this user-friendly cookbook.

$16.95 US • 240 pages • 7.5 x 9-inch quality paperback • ISBN 978-0-7570-0091-1

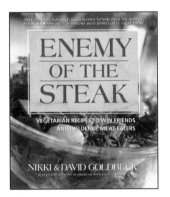

ENEMY OF THE STEAK
Vegetarian Recipes to Win Friends and Influence Meat-Eaters
Nikki and David Goldbeck

Don't blame vegetarians for starting this. Who said "real food for real people"? Aren't asparagus, carrots, and tomatoes every bit as real as . . . that other food? To answer the call to battle, best-selling authors Nikki and David Goldbeck have created a wonderfully tempting new cookbook that offers a wealth of kitchen-tested recipes— recipes that nourish the body, please the palate, and satisfy even the heartiest of appetites.

Enemy of the Steak first presents basic information on vegetarian cooking and stocking the vegetarian pantry. Then eight great chapters offer recipes for breakfast fare; appetizers and hors d'oeuvres; soups; salads; entrées; side dishes; sauces, toppings, and marinades; and desserts. Throughout the book, the Goldbecks have included practical tips and advice on weight loss, disease prevention, and other important topics. They also offer dozens of fascinating facts about why fruits and veggies are so good for you.

A perfect marriage of nutrition and the art of cooking, *Enemy of the Steak* is for everyone who loves a good healthy meal. Simply put, it's great food for smart people. If you have to take sides, you couldn't be in better company.

$16.95 • 248 pages • 7.5 x 9-inch quality paperback • ISBN 978-0-7570-0273-1

Greens & Grains on the Deep Blue Sea Cookbook
Fabulous Vegetarian Cuisine from the Holistic Holiday at Sea Cruises
Sandy Pukel and Mark Hanna

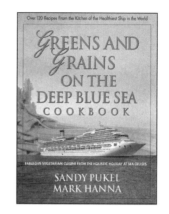

You are invited to come aboard one of America's premier health cruises. Too busy to get away? Even if you can't swim in the ship's pool, you can still enjoy its gourmet cuisine, because natural foods expert Sandy Pukel and master chef Mark Hanna have created *Greens & Grains on the Deep Blue Sea Cookbook*—a titanic collection of the most popular vegetarian dishes served aboard the Holistic Holiday at Sea cruises.

Each of the book's more than 120 recipes is designed to provide not only great taste, but also maximum nutrition. Choose from among an innovative selection of taste-tempting appetizers, soups, salads, entrées, side dishes, and desserts. Easy-to-follow instructions ensure that even novices have superb results. With *Greens & Grains on the Deep Blue Sea Cookbook,* you can enjoy fabulous signature dishes from the Holistic Holiday at Sea cruises in the comfort of your own home.

$16.95 • 160 pages • 7.5 x 9-inch quality paperback • ISBN 978-0-7570-0287-8

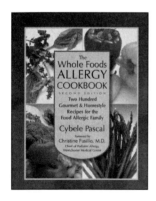

The Whole Foods Allergy Cookbook
Two Hundred Gourmet & Homestyle Recipes for the Food Allergic Family
Cybele Pascal

The Whole Foods Allergy Cookbook is the first cookbook to eliminate all eight allergens responsible for ninety percent of food allergies. Each and every dish offered is free of dairy, eggs, wheat, soy, peanuts, tree nuts, fish, and shellfish. You'll find tempting recipes for breakfast pancakes, breads, and cereals; lunch soups, salads, spreads, and sandwiches; dinner entrées and side dishes; dessert puddings, cupcakes, cookies, cakes, and pies; and even after-school snacks ranging from trail mix to pizza and pretzels. Included is a resource guide to organizations that can supply information and support, as well as a shopping guide for hard-to-find items.

If you thought that allergies meant missing out on nutrition, variety, and flavor, think again. With *The Whole Foods Allergy Cookbook,* you'll have both the wonderful taste you want and the radiant health you deserve.

$18.95 • 240 pages • 8 x 10-inch quality paperback • ISBN 978-1-890612-45-0

THE MISO BOOK
The Art of Cooking with Miso
John and Jan Belleme

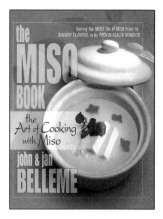

For centuries, the preparation of miso has been considered an art form in Japan. Through a time-honored double-fermentation process, soybeans and grains are transformed into this wondrous food, which is both a flavorful addition to a variety of dishes and a powerful medicinal. Scientific research has supported miso's use as an effective therapeutic aid in the prevention and treatment of heart disease, certain cancers, radiation sickness, and hypertension.

Part One of this comprehensive guide begins with miso basics—its types and uses. A chapter called "Miso Medicine" then details this superfood's healing properties and role in maintaining good health. Easy directions for making miso at home are also found in Part One. Fascinating insets, including the authors' adventures in Japan, where they learned the art of miso-making from a miso master, round out this section. Part Two presents over 140 delectable, healthy recipes in which miso is used in dips, spreads, soups, stews, and so much more.

Whether you are a health-conscious cook in search of healthful foods or you simply are looking for a delicious new take on old favorites, *The Miso Book* may be just what the doctor ordered.

$15.95 • 192 pages • 7.5 x 9-inch quality paperback • ISBN 978-0-7570-0028-7

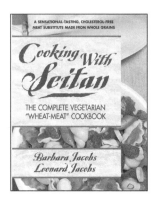

COOKING WITH SEITAN
The Complete Vegetarian "Wheat-Meat" Cookbook
Barbara Jacobs and Leonard Jacobs

Seitan (pronounced *say-tan*) is a spectacular meat substitute with a look, taste, and texture that satisfies the heartiest of appetites. Derived from wheat flour, seitan is naturally nutritious and low in fat, cholesterol, and calories. Perhaps best of all, it is amazingly adaptable and can be seasoned and prepared to fit into any menu.

Cooking with Seitan provides a wonderful introduction to this versatile food. The book explains, step-by-step, how seitan can be made, stored, and used. Also included are over 250 kitchen-tested recipes featuring twists on traditional and international favorites as well as new and imaginative dishes, from salads and appetizers to soups, stews, and even desserts. Whether you want to add to your repertoire of vegetarian dishes or you simply love great food, *Cooking with Seitan* can add a deliciously healthful touch to your menu.

$17.95 • 248 pages • 7.5 x 9-inch quality paperback • ISBN 978-0-7570-0304-2

**For more information about our books,
visit our website at www.squareonepublishers.com**